# STATUS OF HIV/AIDS IN INDIA

# STATUS OF HIV/AIDS IN INDIA

*By*

**A.K. Lobiyal**

**2008**

**CYBER TECH PUBLICATIONS**
4264/3, Ansari Road, Daryaganj, New Delhi-110002 (India)
Ph.: 011-23244078. Fax: 011-23280028
E-Mail: cyberpublicationsdelhi@yahoo.com

# STATUS OF HIV/AIDS IN INDIA

**A.K. Lobiyal**



First Edition 2008



*Published by :*

**G.S. Rawat** for **Cyber Tech Publications**
4264/3, Ansari Road, Daryaganj, New Delhi-110002 (India)
Ph.: 011-23244078. Fax: 011-23280028
E-Mail: cyberpublicationsdelhi@yahoo.com

*Printed at :* **Amit Enterprises**, Maujpur, Delhi, (9810878184)

# Preface

From a few decades back the whole world is confronting with a dreadly disease called HIV/AIDS. An uncurable disease and brings ultimately to death. Medical science is still very far from developing its cure. There is no cure of AIDS only knowledge and prevention can save from it. This disease effects not only men but women and children as well as it is a sexually transmitted disease. Man to women or women to men and then to their children. Many organisations on national and international level are working for the same. Every year and 5th December world AIDS day is celebrated in whole world. Every year it grasps lakhs of precious lines.

The author has mentioned all the facts viz. history and origin and the cases of death of different countries with comparison to India. Mainly India is being focused in this book. A few suggestive measures are also discussed in this book. A brief introduction about the organisations working for curing and importing knowledge and awareness programmes are also mentioned in this book.

The facts and figures relating to AIDS were scattered in magazines, journals and newspapers or data of government author has summed all up in this book for easy perusal of the readers. It is the sincere hope of the author that book will present the deadly face of AIDS and will bring awareness among the people regarding the same.

—*Author*

# Contents

# 1

# Misconceptions about AIDS

The spread of HIV and AIDS has affected millions of people worldwide; According to the "2006 AIDS Epidemic Update", published by the UNAIDS/World Health Organization, there were an estimated 39.5 million people around the world living with HIV, with 4.3 million new HIV infections and 2.9 million deaths from AIDS-related illnesses in 2006. In some regions, there are indications that HIV infection rates have risen by over 50% since 2004. In the wake of this pandemic, a number of misconceptions have arisen surrounding the disease.

## THE RELATIONSHIP BETWEEN HIV AND AIDS

### HIV is the Same as AIDS

This is false. HIV is an acronym for Human Immunodeficiency Virus, and AIDS (Acquired Immune Deficiency Syndrome) is the collection of symptoms, diseases, and infections associated with an acquired deficiency of the immune system. While HIV is almost universally acknowledged as the underlying cause of AIDS, not all HIV-positive individuals have AIDS, as HIV can remain in a latent state for many years.

### HIV does not Cause AIDS

#### *HIV/AIDS Treatment*

**AIDS can be Cured:** There is currently no known cure for AIDS, nor a vaccine for HIV.

Highly Active Anti-Retroviral Therapy (HAART) allows the stabilization of the patient's symptoms and viremia, but it does not cure the patient of HIV or of the symptoms of AIDS. High levels of HIV-1 (often HAART-resistant) return once treatment is stopped. Antiretroviral treatment known as post-exposure prophylaxis reduces the chance of acquiring an HIV infection when administered within 72 hours of exposure to HIV.

It is true that in some cases HIV has been reduced to a survivable chronic condition (an analogy can be made with diabetes-patients with either condition may be treated, leading to a normal quality of life, but this does not constitute a cure). There have been a very small number of cases in which an individual has definitively tested positive and subsequently become negative through treatment or otherwise, but even if these cases are accepted (and there remains debate over their legitimacy), it is not known how this occurred, and it is an extremely rare event in the context of almost fifty million cases of HIV infection worldwide.

### Sexual Intercourse with a Virgin will Cure AIDS

Virgin cleansing is a myth that has occurred since at least the sixteenth century, when Europeans believed that they could rid themselves of a sexually transmitted disease by transferring it to a virgin through sexual intercourse. Although the exact prevalence of this belief is unclear, it is believed to occur worldwide. Sex with an uninfected virgin does not cure an HIV-infected person, and such contact will expose the uninfected individual to HIV, potentially further spreading the disease. This myth has gained considerable notoriety as the perceived reason for certain sexual abuse and child molestation occurrences, especially in Africa.

### Sexual Intercourse with an Animal Will Avoid or Cure AIDS

The National Societies for the Prevention of Cruelty to Animals (NSPCA) in Johannesburg, South Africa, has recorded in 2002 beliefs amongst youths that sex with animals is a means to avoid AIDS or cure it if infected. As with "virgin cure" beliefs, no sexual act can actually cure AIDS. The risk of contracting HIV via sex with animals is small, but the practice has its own health risks. Additionally, sexual intercourse with animals is a criminal offense in a number of countries.

## HIV Antibody Testing is Unreliable

Diagnosis of infection using antibody testing is a well-established technique in medicine. HIV antibody tests exceed the performance of most other infectious disease tests in both sensitivity (the ability of the screening test to give a positive finding when the person tested truly has the disease) and specificity (the ability of the test to give a negative finding when the subjects tested are free of the disease under study). Many current HIV antibody tests have sensitivity and specificity in excess of 96% and are therefore extremely reliable.

Progress in testing methodology has enabled detection of viral genetic material, antigens, and the virus itself in body fluids and cells. While not widely used for routine testing due to high cost and requirements in laboratory equipment, these direct testing techniques have confirmed the validity of the antibody tests. Positive HIV antibody tests are usually followed up by retests and tests for antigens, viral genetic material and the virus itself, providing confirmation of actual infection.

## HIV Infection

AIDS can be spread through casual contact with an HIV infected individual.

One cannot become infected with HIV through day-to-day contact in social settings, schools, or in the workplace; One cannot be infected by shaking someone's hand, by hugging or "dry" kissing someone, by using the same toilet or drinking from the same glass as an HIV-infected person, or by being exposed to coughing or sneezing by an infected person. Saliva carries a negligible viral load, so even open-mouthed kissing is considered a low risk. However, if the infected partner or both of the performers have blood in their mouth due to cuts, open sores, or gum disease, the risk is higher. The CDC has only recorded one case of HIV transmission through kissing, and the Terence Higgins Trust says that this is essentially a no-risk situation.

Other interactions that could theoretically result in person-to-person transmission include caring for nose bleeds, biting, and home health care procedures, yet there are very few recorded incidents of transmission occurring in this way.

## HIV cannot be Transmitted through Oral Sex

While it is agreed that oral sex is a very much lower risk activity-in terms of HIV-infection risk-than vaginal and anal sex, HIV can be transmitted through both insertive and receptive oral sex, when there is contact between semen and the mucous membranes of the mouth. The risk of infection from a single encounter is small, but it increases with frequency of activity according to binomial probability theory. Transmission risk may be elevated in the case of open sores on the genitals and/or mouth, or significant gum disease or bleeding, i.e., when there is direct contact between semen or saliva and breaks in the skin or surface of the mouth. Not sharing hypodermic needles with a seropositive person means one is safe from HIV

Using previously contaminated hypodermic needles or other "works" to divide a drug solution among drug injection partners can spread HIV. Studies in the early-and mid-1980s focused only on sharing needles, but studies beginning in the late-1980s have shown that this message can lead to increased HIV risk of infection because they fail to highlight the risks of infection from sharing the same prep equipment, not just the needles themselves.

## HIV is Transmitted by Mosquitoes

When mosquitoes bite a person, they do not inject the blood of a previous victim into the person they bite next. Mosquitoes do, however, inject saliva into their victims, which may carry diseases such as dengue fever, malaria, yellow fever, or West Nile virus and can infect a bitten person with these diseases. HIV is not transmitted in this manner. On the other hand, a mosquito may have HIV-infected blood in its gut, and if swatted on the skin of a human who then scratches it, transmission may be possible, though this risk is very small, and no cases have yet been identified through this route.

## HIV can Easily be Transmitted to a Person Being Tattooed

Due to the instability of HIV in an open environment, the chances of being infected from the tattooing process are very slim. The virus would be unlikely to survive being exposed to open air on the end of the needle for more than a couple of minutes. Single-use needles and proper precautionary cleaning and sterilization eliminate much of the risk in disease transmission in tattooing. No case of HIV has ever been determined to have been caused by tattooing. Tattooing without proper precautions increases infection risk of several diseases, including HIV and hepatitis.

### HIV can Infect only Homosexual Men and Drug Users

HIV can infect anybody, regardless of any age, sex, ethnicity, or sexual orientation. It is true that anal sex (regardless of the gender of the receptive partner) carries a higher risk of infection than most sex acts, but most penetrative sex acts between any individuals carry some risk. Properly used condoms can reduce this risk.

### An HIV-infected Mother cannot have Children

HIV-infected women are still fertile, although in late stages of HIV disease a pregnant woman may have a higher risk of spontaneous miscarriage. Normally, the risk of transmitting HIV to the unborn child is between 15-30%. However, this may be reduced to just 2-3% if patients carefully follow medical guidelines.

HIV cannot be the cause of AIDS because the body develops a vigorous antibody response to the virus.

This reasoning ignores numerous examples of viruses other than HIV that can be pathogenic after evidence of immunity appears. Measles virus may persist for years in brain cells, eventually causing a chronic neurologic disease despite the presence of antibodies. Viruses such as cytomegalovirus, Herpes simplex virus, and Varicella zoster may be activated after years of latency even in the presence of abundant antibodies. In animals, viral relatives of HIV with long and variable latency periods, such as visna virus in sheep, cause central nervous system damage even after the production of antibodies.

HIV has a well-recognized capacity to mutate to evade the ongoing immune response of the host. Only a small number of CD4+ T cells are infected by HIV, not enough to damage the immune system.

Techniques such as polymerase chain reaction (PCR) have enabled scientists to demonstrate that a much larger proportion of CD4+ T cells are infected than previously realized, particularly in lymphoid tissues. Robert Gallo, a preeminent HIV virologist, suggests that as many as 3% of CD4+ T cells show signs of HIV invasion. Macrophages and other cell types are also infected with HIV and serve as reservoirs for the virus.

Although the fraction of CD4+ T cells that is infected with HIV at any given time is never high (only a small subset of activated cells serve as ideal targets of infection), several groups have shown that rapid cycles of death of infected cells and infection of new target cells occur throughout the course of disease.

Furthermore, like other viruses, HIV is able to suppress the immune system by secreting proteins that interfere with it. For example, HIV's coat protein, gp120, sheds from viral particles and binds to the CD4 receptors of otherwise healthy T cells; this interferes with the normal function of these signalling receptors.

Another HIV protein, Tat, has been demonstrated to suppress T cell activity. This countersurveillance behavior is not significantly different in quality from, say, the influenza viruses, which are well-known to secrete immunosuppressive proteins which can slow down the antiviral immune response.

Infected lymphocytes express the Fas ligand, a cell-surface protein that triggers the death of neighboring uninfected T cells expressing the Fas receptor. This "bystander killing" effect shows that great harm can be caused to the immune system even with a limited number of infected cells.

## HIV TEST

Many people are unaware that they are infected with HIV. Less than 1% of the sexually active urban population in Africa has been tested, and this proportion is even lower in rural populations. Furthermore, only 0.5% of pregnant women attending urban health facilities are counseled, tested or receive their test results. Again, this proportion is even lower in rural health facilities. Therefore, donor blood and blood products used in medicine and medical research are screened for HIV. Typical HIV tests, including the HIV enzyme immunoassay and the Western blot assay, detect HIV antibodies in serum, plasma, oral fluid, dried blood spot or urine of patients.

However, the window period (the time between initial infection and the development of detectable antibodies against the infection) can vary. This is why it can take 3-6 months to seroconvert and test positive. Commercially available tests to detect other HIV antigens, HIV-RNA, and HIV-DNA in order to detect HIV infection prior to the development of detectable antibodies are available.

For the diagnosis of HIV infection these assays are not specifically approved, but are nonetheless routinely used in developed countries.

## SYMPTOMS AND COMPLICATIONS

A generalized graph of the relationship between HIV copies (viral load) and CD4 counts over the average course of untreated HIV infection; any particular individual's disease course may vary considerably.

CD4+ T Lymphocyte count (cells/$mm^3$)

HIV RNA copies per mL of plasma

The symptoms of AIDS are primarily the result of conditions that do not normally develop in individuals with healthy immune systems. Most of these conditions are infections caused by bacteria, viruses, fungi and parasites that are normally controlled by the elements of the immune system that HIV damages. Opportunistic infections are common in people with AIDS. HIV affects nearly every organ system. People with AIDS also have an increased risk of developing various cancers such as Kaposi's sarcoma, cervical cancer and cancers of the immune system known as lymphomas.

Additionally, people with AIDS often have systemic symptoms of infection like fevers, sweats (particularly at night), swollen glands, chills, weakness, and weight loss. After the diagnosis of AIDS is made, the current average survival time with antiretroviral therapy (as of 2005) is estimated to be more than 5 years, but because new treatments continue to be developed and because HIV continues to evolve resistance to treatments, estimates of survival time are likely to continue to change. Without antiretroviral therapy, death normally occurs within a year. Most patients die from opportunistic infections or malignancies associated with the progressive failure of the immune system.

The rate of clinical disease progression varies widely between individuals and has been shown to be affected by many factors such as host susceptibility and immune function health care and co-infections, as well as factors relating to the viral strain. The specific opportunistic infections that AIDS patients develop depend in part on the prevalence of these infections in the geographic area in which the patient lives.

## Major Pulmonary Illnesses

X-ray of Pneumocystis jirovecii caused pneumonia. There is increased white (opacity) in the lower lungs on both sides, characteristic of Pneumocystis pneumonia

- Pneumocystis pneumonia (originally known as Pneumocystis carinii pneumonia, and still abbreviated as PCP, which now stands for Pneumocystis pneumonia) is relatively rare in healthy, immunocompetent people, but common among HIV-infected individuals. It is caused by Pneumocystis jirovecii. Before the advent of effective diagnosis, treatment and routine prophylaxis in Western countries, it was a common immediate cause of death. In developing countries, it is still one of the first indications of AIDS in untested individuals, although it does not generally occur unless the CD4 count is less than 200 per μL.
- Tuberculosis (TB) is unique among infections associated with HIV because it is transmissible to immunocompetent people via the respiratory route, is easily treatable once identified, may occur in early-stage HIV disease, and is preventable with drug therapy. However, multidrug resistance is a potentially serious problem. Even though its incidence has declined because of the use of directly observed therapy and other improved

practices in Western countries, this is not the case in developing countries where HIV is most prevalent. In early-stage HIV infection (CD4 count >300 cells per μL), TB typically presents as a pulmonary disease. In advanced HIV infection, TB often presents atypically with extrapulmonary (systemic) disease a common feature. Symptoms are usually constitutional and are not localized to one particular site, often affecting bone marrow, bone, urinary and gastrointestinal tracts, liver, regional lymph nodes, and the central nervous system. Alternatively, symptoms may relate more to the site of extrapulmonary involvement.

### Major Gastro-intestinal Illnesses

- Esophagitis is an inflammation of the lining of the lower end of the esophagus (gullet or swallowing tube leading to the stomach). In HIV infected individuals, this is normally due to fungal (candidiasis) or viral (herpes simplex-1 or cytomegalovirus) infections. In rare cases, it could be due to mycobacteria.
- Unexplained chronic diarrhea in HIV infection is due to many possible causes, including common bacterial (Salmonella, Shigella, Listeria, Campylobacter, or Escherichia coli) and parasitic infections; and uncommon opportunistic infections such as cryptosporidiosis, microsporidiosis, Mycobacterium avium complex (MAC) and cytomegalovirus (CMV) colitis. In some cases, diarrhea may be a side effect of several drugs used to treat HIV, or it may simply accompany HIV infection, particularly during primary HIV infection. It may also be a side effect of antibiotics used to treat bacterial causes of diarrhea (common for Clostridium difficile). In the later stages of HIV infection, diarrhea is thought to be a reflection of changes in the way the intestinal tract absorbs nutrients, and may be an important component of HIV-related wasting.

### Major Neurological Illnesses

- Toxoplasmosis is a disease caused by the single-celled parasite called Toxoplasma gondii; it usually infects the brain causing toxoplasma encephalitis but it can infect and cause disease in the eyes and lungs.

- Progressive multifocal leukoencephalopathy (PML) is a demyelinating disease, in which the gradual destruction of the myelin sheath covering the axons of nerve cells impairs the transmission of nerve impulses. It is caused by a virus called JC virus which occurs in 70% of the population in latent form, causing disease only when the immune system has been severely weakened, as is the case for AIDS patients. It progresses rapidly, usually causing death within months of diagnosis.
- AIDS dementia complex (ADC) is a metabolic encephalopathy induced by HIV infection and fueled by immune activation of HIV infected brain macrophages and microglia which secrete neurotoxins of both host and viral origin. Specific neurological impairments are manifested by cognitive, behavioral, and motor abnormalities that occur after years of HIV infection and is associated with low CD4+ T cell levels and high plasma viral loads. Prevalence is 10-20% in Western countries but only 1-2% of HIV infections in India. This difference is possibly due to the HIV subtype in India.
- Cryptococcal meningitis is an infection of the meninx (the membrane covering the brain and spinal cord) by the fungus Cryptococcus neoformans. It can cause fevers, headache, fatigue, nausea, and vomiting. Patients may also develop seizures and confusion; left untreated, it can be lethal.

## Major HIV-associated Malignancies

Patients with HIV infection have substantially increased incidence of several malignant cancers. This is primarily due to co-infection with an oncogenic DNA virus, especially Epstein-Barr virus (EBV), Kaposi's sarcoma-associated herpesvirus (KSHV), and human papillomavirus (HPV). The following confer a diagnosis of AIDS when they occur in an HIV-infected person.

- Kaposi's sarcoma (KS) is the most common tumor in HIV-infected patients. The appearance of this tumor in young homosexual men in 1981 was one of the first signals of the AIDS epidemic. Caused by a gammaherpes virus called Kaposi's sarcoma-associated herpes virus (KSHV), it often appears as purplish nodules on the skin, but can affect other organs, especially the mouth, gastrointestinal tract, and lungs.

- High-grade B cell lymphomas such as Burkitt's lymphoma, Burkitt's-like lymphoma, diffuse large B-cell lymphoma (DLBCL), and primary central nervous system lymphoma present more often in HIV-infected patients. These particular cancers often foreshadow a poor prognosis. In some cases these lymphomas are AIDS-defining. Epstein-Barr virus (EBV) or KSHV cause many of these lymphomas.
- Cervical cancer in HIV-infected women is considered AIDS-defining. It is caused by human papillomavirus (HPV).

In addition to the AIDS-defining tumors listed above, HIV-infected patients are at increased risk of certain other tumors, such as Hodgkin's disease and anal and rectal carcinomas. However, the incidence of many common tumors, such as breast cancer or colon cancer, does not increase in HIV-infected patients. In areas where HAART is extensively used to treat AIDS, the incidence of many AIDS-related malignancies has decreased, but at the same time malignant cancers overall have become the most common cause of death of HIV-infected patients.

### Other Opportunistic Infections

AIDS patients often develop opportunistic infections that present with non-specific symptoms, especially low-grade fevers and weight loss. These include infection with Mycobacterium avium-intracellulare and cytomegalovirus (CMV). CMV can cause colitis, as described above, and CMV retinitis can cause blindness. Penicilliosis due to Penicillium marneffei is now the third most common opportunistic infection (after extrapulmonary tuberculosis and cryptococcosis) in HIV-positive individuals within the endemic area of Southeast Asia.

## Transmission and Prevention

*Estimated per act risk for acquisition of HIV by exposure route*

| Exposure Route | Estimated infections per 10,000 exposures to an infected source |
|---|---|
| Blood Transfusion | 9,000 |
| Childbirth | 2,500 |
| Needle-sharing injection drug use | 67 |
| Receptive anal intercourse* | 50 |
| Percutaneous needle stick | 30 |
| Receptive penile-vaginal intercourse* | 10 |
| Insertive anal intercourse* | 6.5 |
| Insertive penile-vaginal intercourse* | 5 |
| Receptive oral intercourse* | 1§ |
| Insertive oral intercourse* | 0.5§ |

* assuming no condom use§ Source refers to oral intercourse performed on a man

The three main transmission routes of HIV are sexual contact, exposure to infected body fluids or tissues, and from mother to fetus or child during perinatal period. It is possible to find HIV in the saliva, tears, and urine of infected individuals, but there are no recorded cases of infection by these secretions, and the risk of infection is negligible.

### Sexual Contact

The majority of HIV infections are acquired through unprotected sexual relations between partners, one of whom has HIV. Sexual transmission occurs with the contact between sexual secretions of one partner with the rectal, genital or oral mucous membranes of another. Unprotected receptive sexual acts are riskier than unprotected insertive sexual acts, with the risk for transmitting HIV from an infected partner to an uninfected partner through unprotected insertive anal intercourse greater than the risk for transmission through vaginal intercourse or oral sex. Oral sex is not without its risks as HIV is transmissible through both insertive and receptive oral sex. The risk of HIV transmission from exposure to saliva is considerably smaller than the risk from exposure to semen; contrary to popular belief, one would have to swallow gallons of saliva from a carrier to run a significant risk of becoming infected.

Approximately 30% of women in ten countries representing "diverse cultural, geographical and urban/rural settings" report that their first sexual experience was forced or coerced, making sexual violence a key driver of the HIV/AIDS pandemic. Sexual assault greatly increases the risk of HIV transmission as protection is rarely employed and physical trauma to the vaginal cavity frequently occurs which facilitates the transmission of HIV.

Sexually transmitted infections (STI) increase the risk of HIV transmission and infection because they cause the disruption of the normal epithelial barrier by genital ulceration and/or microulceration; and by accumulation of pools of HIV-susceptible or HIV-infected cells (lymphocytes and macrophages) in semen and vaginal secretions. Epidemiological studies from sub-Saharan Africa, Europe and North America have suggested that there is approximately a four times greater risk of becoming infected with HIV in the presence of a genital ulcer such as those caused by syphilis and/or chancroid. There is also a significant though lesser increased risk in the presence of STIs such as gonorrhea, Chlamydial infection and trichomoniasis which cause local accumulations of lymphocytes and macrophages.

Transmission of HIV depends on the infectiousness of the index case and the susceptibility of the uninfected partner. Infectivity seems to vary during the course of illness and is not constant between individuals. An undetectable plasma viral load does not necessarily indicate a low viral load in the seminal liquid or genital secretions. Each 10-fold increment of blood plasma HIV RNA is associated with an 81% increased rate of HIV transmission. Women are more susceptible to HIV-1 infection due to hormonal changes, vaginal microbial ecology and physiology, and a higher prevalence of sexually transmitted diseases. People who are infected with HIV can still be infected by other, more virulent strains.

During a sexual act, only male or female condoms can reduce the chances of infection with HIV and other STDs and the chances of becoming pregnant. The best evidence to date indicates that typical condom use reduces the risk of heterosexual HIV transmission by approximately 80% over the long-term, though the benefit is likely to be higher if condoms are used correctly on every occasion. The effective use of condoms and screening of blood transfusion in North America, Western and Central Europe is credited with contributing to the low rates of AIDS in these regions. Promoting condom use, however, has often proved controversial and difficult. Many religious groups, most noticeably the Roman Catholic Church, have opposed the use of condoms on religious grounds, and have sometimes seen condom promotion as an affront to the promotion of marriage, monogamy and sexual morality. Defenders of the Catholic Church's role in AIDS and general STD prevention state that, while they may be against the use of contraception, they are strong advocates of abstinence outside marriage. This attitude is also found among some health care providers and policy makers in sub-Saharan African nations, where HIV and AIDS prevalence is extremely high. They also believe that the distribution and promotion of condoms is tantamount to promoting sex amongst the youth and sending the wrong message to uninfected individuals. However, no evidence has been produced that promotion of condom use increases sexual promiscuity, and abstinence-only programs have been unsuccessful both in changing sexual behavior and in reducing HIV transmission. Evaluations of several abstinence-only programs in the US showed a negative impact on the willingness of youths to use contraceptives, due to the emphasis on contraceptives' failure rates.

The male latex condom, if used correctly without oil-based lubricants, is the single most effective available technology to reduce the sexual transmission of HIV and other sexually transmitted infections. Manufacturers recommend that oil-based lubricants such as petroleum jelly, butter, and lard not be used with latex condoms, because they dissolve the latex, making the condoms porous. If necessary, manufacturers recommend using water-based lubricants. Oil-based lubricants can however be used with polyurethane condoms. Latex condoms degrade over time, making them porous, which is why condoms have expiration dates. In Europe and the United States, condoms have to conform to European (EC 600) or American (D3492) standards to be considered protective against HIV transmission.

The female condom is an alternative to the male condom and is made from polyurethane, which allows it to be used in the presence of oil-based lubricants. They are larger than male condoms and have a stiffened ring-shaped opening, and are designed to be inserted into the vagina. The female condom contains an inner ring, which keeps the condom in place inside the vagina-inserting the female condom requires squeezing this ring. However, at present availability of female condoms is very low and the price remains prohibitive for many women. Preliminary studies suggest that, where female condoms are available, overall protected sexual acts increase relative to unprotected sexual acts, making them an important HIV prevention strategy that must be scaled-up.

With consistent and correct use of condoms, there is a very low risk of HIV infection. Studies on couples where one partner is infected show that with consistent condom use, HIV infection rates for the uninfected partner are below 1% per year.

The United States government and health organizations both endorse the ABC Approach to lower the risk of acquiring AIDS during sex:

*Abstinence or delay of sexual activity, especially for youth,*

*Being faithful, especially for those in committed relationships,*

*Condom use, for those who engage in risky behavior.*

This approach has been very successful in Uganda, where HIV prevalence has decreased from 15% to 5%. However, more has been done than just this. As Edward Green, a Harvard medical anthropologist, put it, “Uganda has pioneered approaches towards reducing stigma, bringing discussion of sexual behavior out into the open, involving HIV-infected people in public education, persuading individuals and couples to be tested and counseled, improving the status of women, involving religious organizations, enlisting traditional healers, and much more." However, criticism of the ABC approach is widespread because a faithful partner of an unfaithful partner is at risk of contracting HIV and that discrimination against women and girls is so great that they are without voice in almost every area of their lives. Other programs and initiatives promote condom use more heavily. Condom use is an integral part of the CNN Approach. This is:

*Condom use, for those who engage in risky behavior,*

*Needles, use clean ones,*

*Negotiating skills; negotiating safer sex with a partner and empowering women to make smart choices.*

In December 2006, the last of three large, randomized trials confirmed that male circumcision lowers the risk of HIV infection among heterosexual African men by around 50%. It is expected that this intervention will be actively promoted in many of the countries worst affected by HIV, although doing so will involve confronting a number of practical, cultural and attitudinal issues. Some experts fear that a lower perception of vulnerability among circumcised men may result in more sexual risk-taking behavior, thus negating its preventive effects. Furthermore, South African medical experts are concerned that the repeated use of unsterilized blades in the ritual circumcision of adolescent boys may be spreading HIV.

### Exposure to Infected Body Fluids

This transmission route is particularly relevant to intravenous drug users, hemophiliacs and recipients of blood transfusions and blood products. Sharing and reusing syringes contaminated with HIV-infected blood represents a major risk for infection with not only HIV, but also hepatitis B and hepatitis C. Needle sharing is the cause of one third of all new HIV-infections and 50% of hepatitis C infections in North America, China, and Eastern Europe. The risk of being infected with HIV from a single prick with a needle that has been used on an HIV-infected person is thought to be about 1 in 150. Post-exposure prophylaxis with anti-HIV drugs can further reduce that small risk. Health care workers (nurses, laboratory workers, doctors etc) are also concerned, although more rarely. This route can affect people who give and receive tattoos and piercings.

Universal precautions are frequently not followed in both sub-Saharan Africa and much of Asia because of both a shortage of supplies and inadequate training. The WHO estimates that approximately 2.5% of all HIV infections in sub-Saharan Africa are transmitted through unsafe healthcare injections. Because of this, the United Nations General Assembly, supported by universal medical opinion on the matter, has urged the nations of the world to implement universal precautions to prevent HIV transmission in health care settings.

The risk of transmitting HIV to blood transfusion recipients is extremely low in developed countries where improved donor selection and HIV screening is performed. However, according to the WHO, the overwhelming majority of the world's population does not have access to safe blood and "between 5% and 10% of HIV infections worldwide are transmitted through the transfusion of infected blood and blood products".

Medical workers who follow universal precautions or body-substance isolation, such as wearing latex gloves when giving injections and washing the hands frequently, can help prevent infection by HIV.

All AIDS-prevention organizations advise drug-users not to share needles and other material required to prepare and take drugs (including syringes, cotton balls, the spoons, water for diluting the drug, straws, crack pipes, etc). It is important that people use new or properly sterilized needles for each injection. Information on cleaning needles using bleach is available from health care and addiction professionals and from needle exchanges. In some developed countries, clean needles are available free in some cities, at needle exchanges or safe injection sites. Additionally, many nations have decriminalized needle possession and made it possible to buy injection equipment from pharmacists without a prescription.

## Mother-to-child Transmission (MTCT)

The transmission of the virus from the mother to the child can occur in utero during the last weeks of pregnancy and at childbirth. In the absence of treatment, the transmission rate between the mother to the child during pregnancy, labor and delivery is 25%. However, when the mother has access to antiretroviral therapy and gives birth by caesarean section, the rate of transmission is just 1%. A number of factors influence the risk of infection, particularly the viral load of the mother at birth (the higher the load, the higher the risk). Breastfeeding increases the risk of transmission by 10-15%. This risk depends on clinical factors and may vary according to the pattern and duration of breast-feeding.

Studies have shown that antiretroviral drugs, caesarean delivery and formula feeding reduce the chance of transmission of HIV from mother to child. Current recommendations state that when replacement feeding is acceptable, feasible, affordable, sustainable and safe, HIV-infected mothers should avoid breast-feeding their infant. However, if this is not the case, exclusive breast-feeding is recommended during the first months of life and discontinued as soon as possible. In 2005, around 700,000 children under 15 contracted HIV, mainly through MTCT, with 630,000 of these infections occurring in Africa. Of the estimated 2.3 million [1.7-3.5 million] children currently living with HIV, 2 million (almost 90%) live in sub-Saharan Africa.

Prevention strategies are well known in developed countries, however, recent epidemiological and behavioral studies in Europe and North America have suggested that a substantial minority of young people continue to engage in high-risk practices and that despite HIV/AIDS knowledge, young people underestimate their own risk of becoming infected with HIV. However, transmission of HIV between intravenous drug users has clearly decreased, and HIV transmission by blood transfusion has become quite rare in developed countries.

## Treatment

There is currently no vaccine or cure for HIV or AIDS. The only known methods of prevention are based on avoiding exposure to the virus or, failing that, an antiretroviral treatment directly after a highly significant exposure, called post-exposure prophylaxis (PEP). PEP has a very demanding four week schedule of dosage. It also has very unpleasant side effects including diarrhea, malaise, nausea and fatigue.

Current treatment for HIV infection consists of highly active antiretroviral therapy, or HAART. This has been highly beneficial to many HIV-infected individuals since its introduction in 1996 when the protease inhibitor-based HAART initially became available. Current optimal HAART options consist of combinations (or "cocktails") consisting of at least three drugs belonging to at least two types, or "classes," of anti-retroviral agents. Typical regimens consist of two nucleoside analogue reverse transcriptase inhibitors (NARTIs or NRTIs) plus either a protease inhibitor or a non-nucleoside reverse transcriptase inhibitor (NNRTI). Because HIV disease progression in children is more rapid than in adults, and laboratory parameters are less predictive of risk for disease progression, particularly for young infants, treatment recommendations are more aggressive for children than for adults. In developed countries where HAART is available, doctors assess the viral load, rapidity in CD4 decline, and patient readiness while deciding when to recommend initiating treatment.

HAART allows the stabilization of the patient's symptoms and viremia, but it neither cures the patient of HIV, nor alleviates the symptoms, and high levels of HIV-1, often HAART resistant, return once treatment is stopped. Moreover, it would take more than the lifetime of an individual to be cleared of HIV infection using HAART. Despite this, many HIV-infected individuals have experienced remarkable improvements in their general health and quality of life, which has led to the plummeting of HIV-associated morbidity and mortality. In the absence of HAART, progression from HIV infection to AIDS occurs at a median of between nine to ten years and the median survival time after developing AIDS is only 9.2 months. HAART is thought to increase survival time by between 4 and 12 years. This average reflects the fact that for some patients-and in many clinical cohorts this may be more than fifty percent of patients-HAART achieves far less than optimal results. This is due to a variety of reasons such as medication intolerance/side effects, prior ineffective antiretroviral therapy and infection with a drug-resistant strain of HIV. However, non-adherence and non-persistence with antiretroviral therapy is the major reason most individuals fail to get any benefit from and develop resistance to HAART. The reasons for non-adherence and non-persistence with HAART are varied and overlapping. Major psychosocial issues, such as poor access to medical care, inadequate social supports, psychiatric disease and drug abuse contribute to non-adherence. The complexity of these HAART regimens, whether due to pill number, dosing frequency, meal restrictions or other issues along with side effects that create intentional non-adherence also has a weighty impact. The side effects include lipodystrophy, dyslipidaemia, insulin resistance, an increase in cardiovascular risks and birth defects.

Anti-retroviral drugs are expensive, and the majority of the world's infected individuals do not have access to medications and treatments for HIV and AIDS. Research to improve current treatments includes decreasing side effects of current drugs, further simplifying drug regimens to improve adherence, and determining the best sequence of regimens to manage drug resistance. However, only a vaccine is postulated to be able to halt the pandemic. This is because a vaccine would possibly cost less, thus being affordable for developing countries, and would not require daily treatments. However, after over 20 years of research, HIV-1 remains a difficult target for a vaccine.

A number of studies have shown that measures to prevent opportunistic infections can be beneficial when treating patients with HIV infection or AIDS. Vaccination against hepatitis A and B is advised for patients who are not infected with these viruses and are at risk of becoming infected. Patients with substantial immunosuppression are also advised to receive prophylactic therapy for Pneumocystis pneumonia (PCP), and many patients may benefit from prophylactic therapy for toxoplasmosis and Cryptococcus meningitis as well. Daily multivitamin and mineral supplements have been found to reduce HIV disease progression among men and women. This could become an important low-cost intervention provided during early HIV disease to prolong the time before antiretroviral therapy is required.

Various forms of alternative medicine have been used to treat symptoms or alter the course of the disease. In the first decade of the epidemic when no useful conventional treatment was available, a large number of people with AIDS experimented with alternative therapies. The definition of "alternative therapies" in AIDS has changed since that time. Then, the phrase often referred to community-driven treatments, untested by government or pharmaceutical company research, that some hoped would directly suppress the virus or stimulate immunity against it. Examples of alternative medicine that people hoped would improve their symptoms or their quality of life include massage, stress management, herbal and flower remedies such as boxwood, and acupuncture; when used with conventional treatment, many now refer to these as "complementary" approaches. Despite the widespread use of complementary and alternative medicine by people living with HIV/AIDS, the effectiveness of these therapies has not been established.

**Epidemiology**

Prevalence of HIV among adults per country at the end of 2005.

15-50% 5-15% 1-5% 0.5-1.0% 0.1-0.5% < 0.1% no data

UNAIDS and the WHO estimate that AIDS has killed more than 25 million people since it was first recognized in 1981, making it one of the most destructive epidemics in recorded history. Despite recent, improved access to antiretroviral treatment and care in many regions of the world, the AIDS epidemic claimed an estimated 2.8 million (between 2.4 and 3.3 million) lives in 2005 of which more than half a million (570,000) were children.

Globally, between 33.4 and 46 million people currently live with HIV. In 2005, between 3.4 and 6.2 million people were newly infected and between 2.4 and 3.3 million people with AIDS died, an increase from 2003 and the highest number since 1981.

Sub-Saharan Africa remains by far the worst affected region, with an estimated 21.6 to 27.4 million people currently living with HIV. Two million [1.5-3.0 million] of them are children younger than 15 years of age. More than 64% of all people living with HIV are in sub-Saharan Africa, as are more than three quarters (76%) of all women living with HIV. In 2005, there were 12.0 million [10.6-13.6 million] AIDS orphans living in sub-Saharan Africa 2005. South & South East Asia are second worst affected with 15%. AIDS accounts for the deaths of 500,000 children in this region. Two-thirds of HIV/AIDS infections in Asia occur in India, with an estimated 5.7 million infections (estimated 3.4-9.4 million) (0.9% of population), surpassing South Africa's estimated 5.5 million (4.9-6.1 million) (11.9% of population) infections, making it the country with the highest number of HIV infections in the world. In the 35 African nations with the highest prevalence, average life expectancy is 48.3 years-6.5 years less than it would be without the disease.

The latest evaluation report of the World Bank's Operations Evaluation Department assesses the effectiveness of the World Bank's country-level HIV/AIDS assistance, defined as policy dialogue, analytic work, and lending, with the explicit objective of reducing the scope or impact of the AIDS epidemic. This is the first comprehensive evaluation of the World Bank's HIV/AIDS support to countries, from the beginning of the epidemic through mid-2004. Because the Bank's assistance is for implementation of government programs by government, it provides important insights on how national AIDS programs can be made more effective.

The development of HAART as effective therapy for HIV infection and AIDS has substantially reduced the death rate from this disease in those areas where it is widely available. This has created the misperception that the disease has gone away. In fact, as the life expectancy of persons with AIDS has increased in countries where HAART is widely used, the number of persons living with AIDS has increased substantially. In the United States, the number of persons with AIDS increased from about 35,000 in 1988 to over 220,000 in 1996.

In Africa, the number of MTCT and the prevalence of AIDS is beginning to reverse decades of steady progress in child survival. Countries such as Uganda are attempting to curb the MTCT epidemic by offering VCT (voluntary counseling and testing), PMTCT (prevention of mother-to-child transmission) and ANC (ante-natal care) services, which include the distribution of antiretroviral therapy.

## Economic Impact

HIV and AIDS retard economic growth by destroying human capital. UNAIDS has predicted outcomes for sub-Saharan Africa to the year 2025. These range from a plateau and eventual decline in deaths beginning around 2012 to a catastrophic continual growth in the death rate with potentially 90 million cases of infection.

Without proper nutrition, health care and medicine that is available in developed countries, large numbers of people in these countries are falling victim to AIDS. They will not only be unable to work, but will also require significant medical care. The forecast is that this will likely cause a collapse of economies and societies in the region. In some heavily infected areas, the epidemic has left behind many orphans cared for by elderly grandparents.

The increased mortality in this region will result in a smaller skilled population and labor force. This smaller labor force will be predominantly young people, with reduced knowledge and work experience leading to reduced productivity. An increase in workers' time off to look after sick family members or for sick leave will also lower productivity. Increased mortality will also weaken the mechanisms that generate human capital and investment in people, through loss of income and the death of parents. By killing off mainly young adults, AIDS seriously weakens the taxable population, reducing the resources available for public expenditures such as education and health services not related to AIDS resulting in increasing pressure for the state's finances and slower growth of the economy. This results in a slower growth of the tax base, an effect that will be reinforced if there are growing expenditures on treating the sick, training (to replace sick workers), sick pay and caring for AIDS orphans. This is especially true if the sharp increase in adult mortality shifts the responsibility and blame from the family to the government in caring for these orphans.

On the level of the household, AIDS results in both the loss of income and increased spending on healthcare by the household. The income effects of this lead to spending reduction as well as a substitution effect away from education and towards healthcare and funeral spending. A study in Côte d'Ivoire showed that households with an HIV/AIDS patient spent twice as much on medical expenses as other households.

UNAIDS, WHO and the United Nations Development Programme have documented a correlation between the decreasing life expectancies and the lowering of gross national product in many African countries with prevalence rates of 10% or more. Indeed, since 1992 predictions that AIDS would slow economic growth in these countries have been published. The degree of impact depended on assumptions about the extent to which illness would be funded by savings and who would be infected. Conclusions reached from models of the growth trajectories of 30 sub-Saharan economies over the period 1990-2025 were that the economic growth rates of these countries would be between 0.56 and 1.47% lower. The impact on gross domestic product (GDP) per capita was less conclusive. However, in 2000, the rate of growth of Africa's per capita GDP was in fact reduced by 0.7% per year from 1990-1997 with a further 0.3% per year lower in countries also affected by malaria. The forecast now is that the growth of GDP for these countries will undergo a further reduction of between 0.5 and 2.6% per annum. However, these estimates may be an underestimate, as they do not look at the effects on output per capita.

Many governments in sub-Saharan Africa denied that there was a problem for years, and are only now starting to work towards solutions. Underfunding is a problem in all areas of HIV prevention when compared to even conservative estimates of the problems.

The launching of the world's first official HIV/AIDS Toolkit in Zimbabwe on October 3, 2006 is a product of collaborative work between the International Federation of Red Cross and Red Crescent Societies, World Health Organization and the Southern Africa HIV/AIDS Information Dissemination Service. It is for the strengthening of people living with HIV/AIDS and nurses by minimal external support. The package, which is in form of eight modules focusing on basic facts about HIV and AIDS, was pre-tested in Zimbabwe in March 2006 to determine its adaptability. It disposes, among other things, categorized guidelines on clinical management, education and counseling of AIDS victims at community level.

The Copenhagen Consensus is a project that seeks to establish priorities for advancing global welfare using methodologies based on the theory of welfare economics. The participants are all economists, with the focus of the project being a rational prioritization based on economic analysis. The project is based on the contention that, in spite of the billions of dollars spent on global challenges by the United Nations, the governments of wealthy nations, foundations, charities, and non-governmental organizations, the money spent on problems such as malnutrition and climate change is not sufficient to meet many internationally-agreed targets. The highest priority was assigned to implementing new measures to prevent the spread of HIV and AIDS. The economists estimated that an investment of $27 billion could avert nearly 30 million new infections by 2010.

**Stigma**

AIDS stigma exists around the world in a variety of ways, including ostracism, rejection, discrimination and avoidance of HIV infected people; compulsory HIV testing without prior consent or protection of confidentiality; violence against HIV infected individuals or people who are perceived to be infected with HIV; and the quarantine of HIV infected individuals. Stigma-related violence or the fear of violence prevents many people from seeking HIV testing, returning for their results, or securing treatment, possibly turning what could be a manageable chronic illness into a death sentence and perpetuating the spread of HIV.

AIDS stigma has been further divided into the following three categories:

1. Instrumental AIDS stigma-a reflection of the fear and apprehension that are likely to be associated with any deadly and transmissible illness.
2. Symbolic AIDS stigma-the use of HIV/AIDS to express attitudes toward the social groups or lifestyles perceived to be associated with the disease.

3. Courtesy AIDS stigma-stigmatization of people connected to the issue of HIV/AIDS or HIV-positive people.

Often, AIDS stigma is expressed in conjunction with one or more other stigmas, particularly those associated with homosexuality, bisexuality, promiscuity, and intravenous drug use. In many developed countries, there is an association between AIDS and homosexuality or bisexuality, and this association is correlated with higher levels of sexual prejudice such as anti-homosexual attitudes. There is also a perceived association between all male-male sexual behavior and AIDS, even sex between two uninfected men. Those most likely to hold misconceptions about HIV transmission and to harbor HIV/AIDS stigma are people with high levels of religiosity, conservative political ideology and less educated people.

### Alternative Hypotheses

A small minority of scientists and activists question the connection between HIV and AIDS, the existence of HIV itself, or the validity of current testing and treatment methods. These claims are considered baseless by the vast majority of the scientific community. The medical community argues that so-called "AIDS dissidents" selectively ignore evidence in favor of HIV's role in AIDS and irresponsibly pose a threat to public health by discouraging HIV testing and proven treatments.

AIDS dissidents assert that the current mainstream approach to AIDS, based on HIV causation, has resulted in inaccurate diagnoses, psychological terror, toxic treatments, and a squandering of public funds. Dissident views have been examined and widely rejected, and are considered pseudoscience by the mainstream scientific community.

## PRINCIPLES

### Screening Donor Blood and Cellular Products

Tests selected to screen donor blood and tissue must provide a high degree of confidence that HIV is not present (that is, a high sensitivity). A combination of antibody, antigen and nucleic acid tests are used by blood banks in Western countries.

The World Health Organization estimated that, as of 2000, inadequate blood screening had resulted in 1 million new HIV infections worldwide. In the USA, most blood donations are screened with an ELISA test for HIV-1 and HIV-2, as well as a nucleic acid test. These diagnostic tests are combined with careful donor selection. As of 2001, the risk of transfusion-acquired HIV in the U.S. was approximately one in 2.5 million for each transfusion.

## Diagnosis of HIV Infection

Tests used for the diagnosis of HIV infection in a particular person require a high degree of both sensitivity and specificity. In the United States, this is achieved using an algorithm combining two tests for HIV antibodies. If antibodies are detected by an initial test based on the ELISA method, then a second test using the Western blot procedure determines the size of the antigens in the test kit binding to the antibodies. The combination of these two methods is highly accurate.

## Human Rights

The UNAIDS/WHO policy statement on HIV Testing states that conditions under which people undergo HIV testing must be anchored in a human rights approach which pays due respect to ethical principles. According to these principles, the conduct of HIV testing of individuals must be:

- Confidential
- Accompanied by counseling
- Conducted with the informed consent of the person being tested

## Antibody Tests

HIV antibody tests are specifically designed for routine diagnostic testing of adults; these tests are inexpensive and extremely accurate.

## Window Period

Antibody tests may give false negative results during the window period, an interval of three weeks to six months between the time of HIV infection and the production of measurable antibodies to HIV (so-called seroconversion). Most people develop detectable antibodies approximately 30 days after infection, although some seroconvert later. The vast majority of people (99%) have detectable antibodies by three months after HIV infection; a six-month window is extremely rare with modern antibody testing. During the window period, an infected person can transmit HIV to others although their HIV infection may not be detectable with an antibody test. Antiretroviral therapy du ing the window period can delay the formation of antibodies and extend the window period beyond 12 months. Antibody tests may also yield false negative results in patients with X-linked agammaglobulinemia; other diagnostic tests should be used in such patients.

Three instances of delayed HIV seroconversion occurring in Health-care workers have been reported; in these instances, the Health-care workers tested negative for HIV antibodies greater than 6 months postexposure but were seropositive within 12 months after the exposure. DNA sequencing confirmed the source of infection in one instance. Two of the delayed seroconversions were associated with simultaneous exposure to hepatitis C virus (HCV). In one case, co-infection was associated with a rapidly fatal HCV disease course; however, it is not known whether HCV directly influences the risk for or course of HIV infection or is a marker for other exposure-related factors.

## ELISA

The ELISA test, or the enzyme immunoassay (EIA), was the first screening test commonly employed for HIV. It has a high sensitivity.

In an ELISA test, a person's serum is diluted 400-fold and applied to a plate to which HIV antigens have been attached. If antibodies to HIV are present in the serum, they may bind to these HIV antigens. The plate is then washed to remove all other components of the serum. A specially prepared "secondary antibody"-an antibody that binds to human antibodies-is then applied to the plate, followed by another wash. This secondary antibody is chemically linked in advance to an enzyme. Thus the plate will contain enzyme in proportion to the amount of secondary antibody bound to the plate. A substrate for the enzyme is applied, and catalysis by the enzyme leads to a change in color or fluorescence. ELISA results are reported as a number; the most controversial aspect of this test is determining the "cut-off" point between a positive and negative result.

### Western Blot

In the Western blot procedure, HIV-infected cells are opened and the proteins within are placed into a slab of gel, to which an electrical current is applied. Different proteins will move with different velocities in this field, depending on their size, while their electrical charge is leveled by a substance called sodium lauryl sulfate. Once the proteins are well-separated, they are transferred to a membrane and the procedure continues similar to an ELISA: the person's diluted serum is applied to the membrane and antibodies in the serum may attach to some of the HIV proteins. Antibodies which do not attach are washed away, and enzyme-linked antibodies with the capability to attach to the person's antibodies determine to which HIV proteins the person has antibodies.

There are no universal criteria for interpreting the Western blot test: the number of viral bands which must be present may vary. If no viral bands are detected, the result is negative. If at least one viral band for each of the GAG, POL, and ENV gene-product groups are present, the result is positive. The three-gene-product approach to Western blot interpretation has not been adopted for public health or clinical practice. Tests in which less than the required number of viral bands are detected are reported as indeterminate: a person who has an indeterminate result should be retested, as later tests may be more conclusive. Almost all HIV-infected persons with indeterminate Western-Blot results will develop a positive result when tested in one month; persistently indeterminate results over a period of six months suggests the results are not due to HIV infection. In a generally healthy low-risk population, indeterminate results on Western blot occur on the order of 1 in 5,000 patients.

**Rapid or Point-of-care Tests**

Rapid Antibody Tests are qualitative immunoassays intended for use as a point-of-care test to aid in the diagnosis of HIV infection. These tests should be used in conjunction with the clinical status, history, and risk factors of the person being tested. The specificity of Rapid Antibody Tests in low-risk populations has not been evaluated. These tests should be used in appropriate multi-test algorithms designed for statistical validation of rapid HIV test results.

If no antibodies to HIV are detected, this does not mean the person has not been infected with HIV. It may take several months after HIV infection for the antibody response to reach detectable levels, during which time rapid testing for antibodies to HIV will not be indicative of true infection status. A comprehensive risk history and clinical judgement should be considered before concluding that an individual is not infected with HIV.

OraQuick is an antibody test that provides results in 20 minutes. The blood, plasma or oral fluid is mixed in a vial with developing solution, and the results are read from a sticklike testing device.

Orasure is an HIV test which uses mucosal transudate from the tissues of cheeks and gums. It is an antibody test which first employs ELISA, then Western Blot.

There is also a urine test; it employs both the ELISA and the Western Blot method.

Home Access Express HIV-1 Test is a FDA-approved home test: the patient collects a drop of blood and mails the sample to a laboratory; the results are obtained over the phone.

There have been a number of cases of fraudulent tests being sold via mail order or the Internet to the general public. In 1997, a California man was indicted on mail fraud and wire charges for selling supposed home test kits. In 2004, the US Federal Trade Commission asked Federal Express and US Customs to confiscate shipments of the Discreet home HIV test kits, produced by Gregory Stephen Wong of Vancouver, BC. In February 2005, the US FDA issued a warning against using the rapid HIV test kits and other home use kits marketed by Globus Media of Montreal Canada.

**Interpreting Antibody Tests**

ELISA testing alone cannot be used to diagnose HIV, even if the test suggests a high probability that antibody to HIV-1 is present. In the United States, such ELISA results are not reported as "positive" unless confirmed by a Western Blot.

The ELISA antibody tests were developed to provide a high level of confidence that donated blood was NOT infected with HIV. It is therefore not possible to conclude that blood rejected for transfusion because of a positive ELISA antibody test is in fact infected with HIV. Sometimes, retesting the donor in several months will produce a negative ELISA antibody test. This is why a confirmatory Western Blot is always used before reporting a "positive" HIV test result.

False positive results due to factors unrelated to exposure to HIV are found more often with the ELISA test than with the Western Blot. False positives can be caused by antibodies to viruses other than HIV, antibodies produced by pregnancy, and other medical conditions such as recent acute illnesses, influenza vaccinations and allergies. A false positive result does not indicate a condition of significant risk to health. When the ELISA test is combined with Western Blot, the rate of false positives is extremely low, and diagnostic accuracy is very high.

**Accuracy of HIV Testing**

The evidence regarding the risks and benefits of HIV screening was reviewed in July 2005 by the U.S. Preventive Services Task Force. The authors concluded that:...the use of repeatedly reactive enzyme immunoassay followed by confirmatory Western blot or immunofluorescent assay remains the standard method for diagnosing HIV-1 infection.

A large study of HIV testing in 752 U.S. laboratories reported a sensitivity of 99.7% and specificity of 98.5% for enzyme immunoassay, and studies in U.S. blood donors reported specificities of 99.8% and greater than 99.99%. With confirmatory Western blot, the chance of a false-positive identification in a low-prevalence setting is about 1 in 250 000 (95% CI, 1 in

173 000 to 1 in 379 000). Other studies have confirmed the accuracy of current methods of HIV testing in the United States, reporting false-positive rates of 0.0004% to 0.0007% and false-negative rates of 0.003% in the general population.

## Antigen Tests

The p24 antigen test detects the presence of the p24 protein of HIV (also known as CA), a major core protein of the virus. Monoclonal antibodies specific to the p24 protein are mixed with the person's blood. Any p24 protein in the person's blood will stick to the monoclonal antibody and enzyme-linked antibody to the monoclonal antibodies to p24 causes a color change if p24 was present in the sample.

This test is no longer used routinely in the US or the EU to screen blood donations since the objective was to reduce the risk of false negatives in the window period. Nucleic acid testing (NAT) is more effective for this purpose, and p24 antigen testing is no longer indicated if a NAT test is performed. The p24 antigen test is not useful for general diagnostics, as it has very low sensitivity and only works during a certain time period after infection before the body produces antibodies to the p24 protein.

## Nucleic Acid based Tests (NAT)

Nucleic-acid-based tests amplify and detect a 142-base target sequence located in a highly conserved region of the HIV gag gene. Since 2001, donated blood in the United States has been screened with nucleic-acid-based tests, shortening the window period between infection and detectability of disease to about 12 days. Since these tests are relatively expensive, the blood is screened by first pooling some 10-20 samples and testing these together; if the pool tests positive, each sample is retested individually. A different version of this test is intended for use in conjunction with clinical presentation and other laboratory markers of disease progress for the management of HIV-1-infected patients.

In the RT-PCR test, viral RNA is extracted from the patient's plasma and is treated with reverse transcriptase so that the RNA of the virus is transcribed into DNA. The polymerase chain reaction (PCR) is then applied, using two primers thought to be unique to the virus's genome. After the PCR amplification process is complete, the resulting amplified segments bind to specific oligonucleotides bound to the vessel wall and are then made visible with a probe bound to an enzyme. The amount of virus in the sample can be quantified with sufficient accuracy to detect three-fold changes.

In the Quantiplex bDNA or branched DNA test, plasma is centrifugated to concentrate the virus, which is then opened to release its RNA. Special oligonucleotides are added which bind to viral RNA and to certain oligonucleotides bound to the wall of the vessel. In this way, viral RNA is fastened to the wall. Then new oligonucleotides are added which bind at several locations to this RNA; and other oligonucelotides which bind at several locations to those oligonucleotides. This is done to amplify the signal. Finally, oligonucleotides that bind to the last set of oligonucleotides and that are bound to an enzyme are added; the enzyme action causes a color reaction which allows quantification of the viral RNA in the original sample. Monitoring the effects of antiretroviral therapy by serial measurements of plasma HIV-1 RNA with this test has been validated for patients with viral loads greater than 25,000 copies per milliliter.

**Other Tests used in HIV/AIDS Treatment**

The CD4 T-cell count is not an HIV test, but rather a procedure where the number of CD4 T-cells in the blood is determined.

A CD4 count does not check for the presence of HIV. It is used monitor immune system function in HIV-positive people. Declining CD4 T-cell counts are considered to be a marker of progression of HIV infection. In HIV-positive people, AIDS is officially diagnosed when the count drops below 200 cells/μL or when certain opportunistic infections occur. This use of a CD4 count as an AIDS criterion was introduced in 1992; the value of 200 was chosen because it corresponded with a greatly increased likelihood of opportunistic infection. Lower CD4 counts in people with AIDS are indicators that prophylaxis against certain types of opportunistic infections should be instituted.

Low CD4 T-cell counts are associated with a variety of conditions, including many viral infections, bacterial infections, parasitic infections, sepsis, tuberculosis, coccidioidomycosis, burns, trauma, intravenous injections of foreign proteins, malnutrition, over-exercising, pregnancy, normal daily variation, psychological stress, and social isolation. This test is also used occasionally to estimate immune system function for people whose CD4 T cells are impaired for reasons other than HIV infection, which include several blood diseases, several genetic disorders, and the side effects of many chemotherapy drugs. Generally speaking, the lower the number of T cells, the lower the immune system's function will be. Normal CD4 counts are between 500 and 1500 CD4+ T cells/microliter, and the counts may fluctuate in healthy people depending on recent infection status, nutrition, exercise and other factors. Women tend to have somewhat lower counts than men.

## CRITICISMS OF HIV TESTS

HIV tests have been criticized by a number of AIDS dissidents (people who reject the scientific consensus that HIV causes AIDS), including the Perth Group of scientists (led by Eleni Papadopulos-Eleopulos) who question the very existence of HIV. Their arguments rest on issues of specificity, standardisation, reproducibility, and validation. According to scientific consensus, the accuracy of serologic testing has been verified by isolation and culture of HIV and by detection of HIV RNA by PCR, which are widely accepted "gold standards" in microbiology. While the AIDS dissidents focus on individual components of HIV testing, it is generally believed that the combination of ELISA and Western Blot used for the diagnosis of HIV is remarkably accurate, with very low false-positive and-negative rates as described above. The vast majority of scientists believe that the views of AIDS dissidents are based on highly selective analysis of mostly outdated scientific papers; there is broad scientific consensus that HIV is the cause of AIDS.

## RATES OF HIV DISEASE PROGRESSION

Following infection with HIV-1, the rate of clinical disease progression varies between individuals. Factors such as host susceptibility, genetics and immune function (Morgan et al., 2002b), health care and co-infections (Morgan et al., 2002a) as well as viral genetic variability (Campbell et al., 2004) may affect the rate of progression to AIDS.

### Rapid Progressors

A small percentage of HIV-infected individuals rapidly progress to AIDS within four years after primary HIV-infection and are termed Rapid Progressors (RP) (Anzala et al., 1995). Indeed some individuals have been known to progress to AIDS and death within a year after primo-infection. Rapid progression was originally thought to be continent specific, as some studies reported that disease progression is more rapid in Africa (N'Galy et al., 1988; Anzala et al., 1995; Whittle et al., 1992), but others have contested this view (Marlink et a., 1994; French et al., 1999; Morgan et al., 2002).

### Long Term Non-Progressors

Another subset of individuals who are persistently infected with HIV-1, but show no signs of disease progression for over 12 years and remain asymptomatic are classified as Long Term Non-Progressors (LTNP). In these individuals, it seems that HIV-infection has been halted with regard to disease progression over an extended period of time (Buchbinder et al., 1994; Cao et al., 1995; Easterbrook, 1994; Levy, 1993). However, the term LTNP is a misnomer, as it must be noted that progression towards AIDS can occur even after 15 years of stable infection (Harrer et al., 1996). LTNP are not a homogeneous group regarding both viral load and specific immune responses against HIV-1. Some LTNPs are infected with HIV that inefficiently replicates (Deacon et al., 1995; Kirchhoff et al., 1995) whilst others are infected with HIV that is virally fit and replicates normally, but the infected individual has had a strong and broad set of HIV-specific humoral and cell-mediated responses that seems to delay the progression to AIDS. In some cohorts, individuals who experience signs of progression, but whose clinical and laboratory parameters remain stable over long periods of time, are classified as Long Term Survivors (LTS) (Schrager et al., 1994; Campbell et al., 2004).

## Highly Exposed Persistently Seronegative

There is another, smaller percentage of individuals who have been recently identified. These are called Highly Exposed Persistently Seronegative (HEPS). This is a small group of individuals and has been observed only in a group of uninfected HIV-negative prostitutes in Kenya and in The Gambia. When these individuals' PBMCs are stimulated with HIV-1 peptides, they have lymphoproliferative activity and have HIV-1 specific CD8+ CTL activity suggesting that transient infection may have occurred (Clerici et al., 1994; Pinto et al., 1995; Rowland-Jones et al., 1995; Fowke et al., 1996). This does not occur in unexposed individuals. What is interesting, is that the CTL epitope specificity differs between HEPS and HIV positive individuals, and in HEPS, the maintenance of responses appears to be dependent upon persistent exposure to HIV (Kaul et al., 2001).

## Prediction of Progression Rates

During the initial weeks after HIV infection, qualitative differences in the cell-mediated immune response are observed that correlate with different disease progression rates (i.e., rapid progression to WHO stage 4 and the rapid loss of CD4+ T cell levels versus normal to slow progression to WHO stage 4 and the maintenance of CD4+ T cell counts above 500/µl). The appearance of HIV-1-specific CD8+ cytotoxic T cells (CTLs) early after primo-infection has been correlated with the control of HIV-1 viremia (Koup et al., 1994; Borrow et al., 1994). The virus which escapes this CTL response have been found to have mutations in specific CTL epitopes (Philips et al., 1991; Borrow et al., 1997; Price et al., 1997; Rowland-Jones et al., 1992). Individuals with a broad expansion of the V-beta chain of the T cell receptor of CD8+ T cells during primo-infection appear seem to have low levels of virus six to twelve months later, which is predictive of relatively slow disease progression. In contrast, individuals with an expansion of only a single subset of the V-beta chain of the CD8+ T cells are not able to control HIV levels over time, and thus have high levels of virus six to twelve months later (Pantaleo et al., 1997). LTNP's have also been shown to have a vigorous proliferation of circulating activated HIV-1-specific CD4+ T cell (Rosenberg et al., 1997) and CTL response (Rowland-Jones et al., 1999; Dyer et al., 1999) against multiple epitopes with no detectable broadly cross-reactive neutralizing antibodies in the setting of an extremely low viral load (Harrer et al., 1996). However, a few reports have correlated the presence of antibodies against Tat and LTNP status.

### HIV Subtype Variation and Effect on Progression Rates

The HIV-1 subtype that an individual becomes infected with can be a major factor in the rate of progression from sero-conversion to AIDS. Individuals infected with subtypes C, D and G are 8 times more likely to develop AIDS than individuals infected with subtype A (Kanki et al., 1999). In Uganda, where subtypes A and D are most prevalent (Kaleebu et al., 2000), subtype D is associated with faster disease progression compared with subtype A (Kaleebu et al., 2002). Age has also been shown to be a major factor in determining survival and the rate of disease progression, with individuals over 40 years of age at sero-conversion being associated with rapid progression (Koblin et al., 1999; Pezotti et al., 1999; Collaborative Group, 2000; Morgan et al., 2002b).

### Host Genetic Susceptibility

The Centers for Disease Control and Prevention (CDC) has released findings that genes influence susceptibility to HIV infection and progression to AIDS. HIV enters cells through an interaction with both CD4 and a chemokine receptor of the 7 Tm family. They first reviewed the role of genes in encoding chemokine receptors (CCR5 and CCR2) and chemokines (SDF-1). While CCR5 has multiple variants in its coding region, the deletion of a 32-bp segment results in a nonfunctional receptor, thus preventing HIV entry; two copies of this gene provide strong protection against HIV infection, although the protection is not absolute. This gene is found in up to 20% of Europeans but is rare in Africans and Asians. Multiple studies of HIV-infected persons have shown that presence of one copy of this gene delays progression to the condition of AIDS by about 2 years. And it is possible that a person with the CCR5-?32 receptor gene will not be infected with HIV.

## The effect of Co-infections on Progression Rates

Co-infections or immunizations may enhance viral replication by inducing a response and activation of the immune system. This activation facilitates the three key stages of the viral life cycle: entry to the cell; reverse transcription and proviral transcription (Lawn et al., 2001). Chemokine receptors are vital for the entry of HIV into cells. The expression of these receptors is inducible by immune activation caused through infection or immunization, thus augmenting the number of cells that are able to be infected by HIV-1 (Wahl et al., 1998; Juffermans et al., 2001). Both reverse transcription of the HIV-1 genome and the rate of transcription of proviral DNA rely upon the activation state of the cell and are less likely to be successful in quiescent cells. In activated cells there is an increase in the cytoplasmic concentrations of mediators required for reverse transcription of the HIV genome (Zack et al., 1990; Kinoshita et al., 1998). Activated cells also release IFN-alpha which acts on an autocrine and paracrine loop that up-regulates the levels of physiologically active NF-kappa B which activates host cell genes as well as the HIV-1 LTR (Gaynor, 1992; Baeuerle, 1991). The impact of co-infections by micro-organisms such as Mycobacterium tuberculosis can be important in disease progression, particularly for those who have a high prevalence of chronic and recurrent acute infections and poor access to medical care (Blanchard et al., 1997). Often, survival depends upon the initial AIDS-defining illness (Morgan et al., 1997). Co-infection with DNA viruses such as HTLV-1, herpes simplex virus-2, varicella zoster virus and cytomegalovirus may enhance proviral DNA transcription and thus viral load as they may encode proteins that are able to trans-activate the expression of the HIV-1 pro-viral DNA (Gendelman et al., 1986). Frequent exposure to helminth infections, which are endemic in Africa, activates individual immune systems, thereby shifting the cytokine balance away from an initial Th1 cell response against viruses and bacteria which would occur in the uninfected person to a less protective T helper 0/2-type response (Bentwich et al., 1995). HIV-1 also promotes a Th1 to Th0 shift and replicates preferentially in Th2 and Th0 cells (Maggi et al., 1994). This makes the host more susceptible to and less able to cope with infection with HIV-1, bacteria and other viruses.

## HIV VACCINE

An HIV vaccine is a hypothetical vaccine against HIV, the etiological agent of AIDS. As there is no known cure for AIDS, the search for a vaccine has become part of the struggle against the disease.

The urgency of the search for a vaccine against HIV stems from the AIDS-related death toll of over 25 million people since 1981. Indeed, in 2002, AIDS became the primary cause of mortality due to an infectious agent in Africa (UNAIDS, 2004).

Alternative medical treatments to a vaccine do exist. Highly active antiretroviral therapy (HAART) has been highly beneficial to many HIV-infected individuals since its introduction in 1996 when the protease inhibitor-based HAART initially became available. HAART allows the stabilisation of the patient's symptoms and viremia, but they do not cure the patient of HIV, nor of the symptoms of AIDS (Martinez-Picardo et al., 2000). And, importantly, HAART does nothing to prevent the spread of HIV through people with undiagnosed HIV infections. Safer sex measures have also proven insufficient to halt the spread of AIDS in the worst affected countries, despite some success in reducing infection rates. Therefore, a HIV vaccine is generally considered as the most likely, perhaps the only way by which the AIDS pandemic can be halted. However, after over 20 years of research, HIV-1 remains a difficult target for a vaccine.

### Difficulties in Developing an HIV Vaccine

In 1984, after the confirmation of the etiological agent of AIDS by Prof. Robert Gallo, the United States Health and Human Services Secretary Margaret Heckler declared that a vaccine would be available within two years (Associated Press, 1984). However, the classical vaccination approaches that have been successful in the control of various viral diseases by priming the adaptive immunity to recognise the viral envelope proteins have failed in the case of HIV-1, as the epitopes of the viral envelope are too variable. Furthermore, the functionally important epitopes of the gp120 protein are masked by glycosylation, trimerisation and receptor-induced conformational changes making it difficult to block with neutralising antibodies. In February 2003, Vaxgen announced that their AIDSVAX vaccine was a failure in North America as there was not a statistically significant reduction of HIV infection within the study population (Francis et al., 2003). In November 2003, it also failed clinical trials in Thailand for the same reason. These vaccines both targeted gp120 and were specific for the geographical regions (Billich et al., 2001).

The ineffectiveness of previously developed vaccines primarily stems from two related factors. First, HIV is highly mutable. Because of the virus' ability to rapidly respond to selective pressures imposed by the immune system, the population of virus in an infected individual typically evolves so that it can evade the two major arms of the adaptive immune system; humoral (antibody-mediated) and systemic (mediated by T cells) immunity. Second, HIV isolates are themselves highly variable. HIV can be categorized into multiple clades and subtypes with a high degree of genetic divergence. Therefore, the immune responses raised by any vaccine need to be broad enough to account for this variability. Any vaccine that lacks this breadth is unlikely to be effective.

The typical animal model for vaccine research is the monkey, often the macaque. The monkeys can be infected with SIV or the chimeric SHIV for research purposes. However, the well-proven route of trying to induce neutralizing antibodies by vaccination has stalled because of the great difficulty in stimulating antibodies that neutralise heterologous primary HIV isolates (Poignard et al., 1999). Some vaccines based on the virus envelope have protected chimpanzees or macaques from homologous virus challenge (Berman et al., 1990), but in clinical trials, individuals who were immunised with similar constructs became infected after later exposure to HIV-1 (Connor et al., 1998).

The human body can defend itself against HIV, as work with monoclonal antibodies (MAb) has proven. That certain individuals can be asymptomatic for decades after infection is encouraging.

## RESEARCH ACHIEVEMENTS

Research supports the contention that a safe and effective vaccine is possible. Vaccines against other diseases where correlates were not known and where there were no ideal animal model have been developed.

Most HIV is transmitted heterosexually, which is known to be less efficient than parenteral exposure. Finally, individuals who become infected with HIV do not succumb to the disease for years even in the absence of anti-retroviral therapy, suggesting that the human immune system is capable of controlling HIV infection partially or temporarily.

Enormous effort has been put into understanding how HIV works; it has produced a number of approaches to vaccination, none of which have been effective. Methods attempted include recombinant proteins, synthetic peptides, recombinant viral vectors, recombinant bacterial vectors, recombinant particles, DNA vaccines to induce production of a specific antigen, and whole-killed and live-attenuated HIV, though these latter two have not progressed into clinical trials in uninfected individuals due to an unfavorable benefit/risk ratio. The role of broadly neutralising antibodies (NAb) is under investigation, although earlier results were discouraging. Vaccines are used to investigate the HIV glycoproteins. Attacks on particular parts of the RNA code of the virus have shown some promise, such as those against the nef gene which regulates viral replication.

On November 16, 2004, researchers at the French Institut Pasteur announced that they had been able to induce antibodies to significantly block HIV from infecting human cells, an achievement hailed as an important step towards an HIV vaccine.

This article or section needs to be updated.Parts of this article or section have been identified as no longer being up to date.Please update the article to reflect recent events, and remove this template when finished.

On November 29, 2004, Wei Lu, Jean-Marie Andrieu, and colleagues at the University of Paris in France and Pernambuco Federal University in Recife, Brazil, tested a vaccine on 18 Brazilian patients whose T-cell counts stopped dropping after getting three under-the-skin injections of the tailor-made vaccine. Novel Vaccine Stops HIV. On December 1, 2004, Swedish media announced that a new vaccine will be tested on

40 volunteers. If the new method is successful, vaccinations will be performed in Tanzania next year.

On March 13, 2005, China announced it began human trials for an AIDS vaccine. 49 volunteers between the ages of 18 and 50 would receive the vaccine.

On April 14, 2006, Atlanta 12 uninfected volunteers are to start getting the newly developed HIV vaccine.

The burden of HIV-related disease and transmission in Africa demands that enhanced efforts be made to treat large numbers of infected people with antiretroviral drugs, despite the cost and the emergence of resistant strains, while effective preventative vaccines are developed. Also, access to care and the development of simplified monitoring schemes for positive and negative treatment effects, as well as effective planning on how to obtain and distribute HIV vaccines needs to be addressed. This will be an important step if a large scale phase III HIV-vaccine trial is to be effective (WHO-UNAIDS, 2001), as this may bypass what we saw with antiretroviral therapy, that drugs were initially widely used in only developed countries.

## Clinical Trials to Date

17 vaccine candidates are in phase I trials and four in phase I/II. There is only one in phase III (the NIH/Department of Defense's ALVAC vCP 1521 canary pox vector/AIDSVAX prime-boost vaccine trial now under way in Thailand).

This article or section needs to be updated.Parts of this article or section have been identified as no longer being up to date.Please update the article to reflect recent events, and remove this template when finished.

Up to May 2000 over 60 phase I/II trials of candidate vaccines had been conducted worldwide. Most initial approaches focused on the HIV envelope protein. At least thirteen different gp120 and gp160 envelope candidates have been evaluated, in the US predominantly through the AIDS Vaccine Evaluation Group. Most research focused on gp120 rather than gp41/gp160, as the latter are generally more difficult to produce and did not initially offer any clear advantage over gp120 forms. Overall, they have been safe and immunogenic in diverse populations, have induced neutralizing antibody in nearly 100% recipients, but rarely induced CD8+ cytotoxic T lymphocytes (CTL). Mammalian derived envelope preparations have been better inducers of neutralizing antibody than candidates produced in yeast and bacteria. Although the vaccination process involved many repeated "booster" injections, it was very difficult to induce and maintain the high anti-gp120 antibody titers necessary to have any hope of neutralizing an HIV exposure.

The availability of several recombinant canarypox vectors has provided interesting results that may prove to be generalizable to other viral vectors. Increasing the complexity of the canarypox vectors by inclusion of more genes/epitopes has increased the percent of volunteers that have detectable CTL to a greater extent than did increasing the dose of the viral vector. Importantly, CTLs from volunteers were able to kill peripheral blood mononuclear cells infected with primary isolates of HIV, suggesting that induced CTLs could have biological significance. In addition, cells from at least some volunteers were able to kill cells infected with HIV from other clades, though the pattern of recognition was not uniform among volunteers. As canarypox is the first candidate HIV vaccine that has induced cross-clade functional CTL responses,

Other strategies that have progressed to phase I trials in uninfected persons include peptides, lipopeptides, DNA, an attenuated Salmonella vector, lipopeptides, p24, etc. Specifically, candidate vaccines that induce one or more of the following are being sought:

- broadly neutralizing antibody against HIV primary isolates;
- cytotoxic T cell responses in a vast majority of recipients;
- strong mucosal immune responses.

On December 13, 2004, a large phase II clinical trial of a novel HIV vaccine began enrolling volunteers at sites in North America, South America, the Caribbean and Australia. The organizers were seeking 3,000 participants. The trial was co-funded by the National Institute of Allergy and Infectious Diseases (NIAID), part of the National Institutes of Health (NIH), and the pharmaceutical company Merck & Co. Inc.

Merck developed the experimental vaccine to stimulate HIV-specific cellular immunity, which prompts the body to produce T cells that kill HIV-infected cells. In previous smaller trials, this vaccine was found to be safe and to induce cellular immune responses against HIV in more than half of volunteers.

The Merck vaccine contains a weakened adenovirus that serves as a carrier for three subtype B HIV genes. Subtype B is the most prevalent HIV subtype in the regions of the study sites. Adenoviruses are among the main causes of upper respiratory tract ailments such as the common cold. Because the vaccine contains only three HIV genes housed in a weakened adenovirus, study participants cannot become infected with HIV or get a respiratory infection from the vaccine.

Organizers expect that it will take approximately one and a half years to fully enroll volunteers into the study. NIAID and Merck expect the trial be completed in four-and-a-half years, with results anticipated in 2009. More information on enrollment can be found at HVTN's Web site.

Novel approaches, including modified vaccinia Ankara (MVA), adeno-associated virus, Venezuelan Equine Encephalitis (VEE) replicons, and codon-optimized DNA have proven to be strong inducers of CTL in macaque models, and have provided at least partial protection in some models. Most of these approaches are, or will soon, enter clinical studies.

## Economics of Vaccine Development

A June 2005 study estimates that $682 million is spent on AIDS vaccine research annually (CITE).

Economic issues with developing an AIDS vaccine include the need for advance purchase commitment (or advance market commitments) because after an AIDS vaccine has been developed, governments and NGOs may be able to bid the price down to marginal cost (CITE).

Conducting trials of HIV vaccines in the countries most affected by the epidemic is a challenge, albeit one that has been successfully met in Thailand. When one or more HIV-1 vaccines is identified, the task will be just beginning. The next step will be ensuring access for populations where the need is the greatest.

Currently, over 60 million people have become infected with HIV-1 and hundreds of millions are at risk. Many of these individuals have little access to medical care, no access to adult vaccinations and live in countries where the per capita expenditure on health care is a few dollars.

Often, HIV-1 is ill understood and stigmatized. Diagnostic tests or algorithms may need to be altered. Education will be needed to convey not only the value but the anticipated limitations of the vaccines, so that other preventive strategies will be maintained. The role of community organizations in maintaining this balance will be critical. Regulatory approvals in numerous countries will be required. The issues in the USA are complex. Internationally, there are greater challenges. If a vaccine has not been demonstrated to be universally effective against every HIV-1 subtype, the standard paradigm of approval in one or more industrialized countries followed years or even decades later by acceptance in and distribution to developing countries will not apply. Both the governments of countries affected by HIV-1 and the international regulatory and health authorities must plan ahead for the advent of an HIV-1 vaccine to avoid unnecessary delays.

HIV-1 vaccines might induce antibody responses that would completely prevent HIV-1 infection by strains of virus that are sufficiently well matched to the vaccine. Unfortunately, HIV-1 evolves continuously both within an individual (the source of infection) and within human populations. Therefore, a vaccinated person might be protected initially, but later encounter a virus against which he or she is not immune. Multivalent vaccines or repeated immunization with an updated vaccine may be required for continued protection. Thus, eventually, one might imagine licensure not of a specific HIV-1 vaccine but of a method for producing the vaccine and its updated versions, somewhat analogous to the annual updates of influenza vaccine.

The scientific challenges involved in discovery of a safe and effective vaccine against HIV-1, although daunting, are only the prelude. The task of developing and deploying a vaccine against HIV-1 will be enormous (i.e. gaining licensure and scaling up to produce vaccine for worldwide distribution, developing distribution methods and establishing purchase mechanisms will require an unprecedented co-operative effort by governments, international agencies, philanthropic organizations and the private sector). Recent recognition of the importance of controlling HIV-1 for public health, economic and political stability has been encouraging and there has been substantial growth in academic, government, nonprofit and pharmaceutical industry vaccine research, but the fight is not over. Stopping the march of the pandemic will conserve economic and human resources needed to care for those already infected. Ending the HIV-1 epidemic is critical to allow economic development and promote political stability in the developing world and to reduce loss of life and suffering worldwide.

### Controversy

Reginald Finger, M.D., M.P.H., a member of the Advisory Committee on Immunization Practices (ACIP) in the U.S., has stated that the Committee would have to carefully consider an HIV vaccine's effects on sexual activity. In an interview with Michael Specter of The New Yorker, he said: "'We would have to look at that closely... With any vaccine for H.I.V., disinhibition... would certainly be a factor, and it is something we will have to pay attention to with a great deal of care.'"

Disinhibition is a "medical term for the absence of fear," in this case, fear of sexual activity.

This article or section needs to be updated.Parts of this article or section have been identified as no longer being up to date.Please update the article to reflect recent events, and remove this template when finished.

Similar controversy has arisen in response to the recent introduction of the HPV vaccine, which prevents infection with certain strains of human papillomavirus, another sexually transmitted disease.

ACIP is an influential government committee linked to the Centers for Disease Control. ACIP is charged with advising the President on prevention of vaccine-related diseases. Dr. Finger's term expired in June, 2006.

# 2

# HIV/AIDS: What is It?

## INTRODUCTION

HIV stands for human immunodeficiency virus. This is the virus that causes AIDS. HIV is different from most other viruses because it attacks the immune system. The immune system gives our bodies the ability to fight infections. HIV finds and destroys a type of white blood cell (T cells or CD4 cells) that the immune system must have to fight disease.

## AIDS

AIDS stands for acquired immunodeficiency syndrome. AIDS is the final stage of HIV infection. It can take years for a person infected with HIV, even without treatment, to reach this stage. Having AIDS means that the virus has weakened the immune system to the point at which the body has a difficult time fighting infections. When someone has one or more of these infections and a low number of T cells, he or she has AIDS. Electron microscope image of HIV, seen as small spheres on the surface of white blood cells.

## ORIGIN OF HIV

First of all the scientists identified a type of chimpanzee in West Africa as the source of HIV infection in humans. The virus most likely jumped to humans when humans hunted these chimpanzees for meat and came into contact with their infected blood. Over several years, the virus slowly spread across Africa and later into other parts of the world.

## HISTORY OF HIV IN THE US

HIV was first identified in the United States in 1981 after a number of gay men started getting sick with a rare type of cancer. It took several years for scientists to develop a test for the virus, to understand how HIV was transmitted between humans, and to determine what people could do to protect themselves. During the early 1980s, as many as 150,000 people became infected with HIV each year. By the early 1990s, this rate had dropped to about 40,000 each year, where it remains today.

AIDS cases began to fall dramatically in 1996, when new drugs became available. Today, more people than ever before are living with HIV/AIDS. CDC estimates that about 1 million people in the United States are living with HIV or AIDS. About one quarter of these people do not know that they are infected: not knowing puts them and others at risk. For more information view the spotlight on 25 years of HIV/AIDS.

## HOW HIV IS AND IS NOT TRANSMITTED?

HIV is a fragile virus. It cannot live for very long outside the body. As a result, the virus is not transmitted through day-to-day activities such as shaking hands, hugging, or a casual kiss. You cannot become infected from a toilet seat, drinking fountain, doorknob, dishes, drinking glasses, food, or pets. You also cannot get HIV from mosquitoes.

HIV is primarily found in the blood, semen, or vaginal fluid of an infected person. HIV is transmitted in 3 main ways:

- Having sex (anal, vaginal, or oral) with someone infected with HIV.
- Sharing needles and syringes with someone infected with HIV.
- Being exposed (fetus or infant) to HIV before or during birth or through breast feeding.

HIV also can be transmitted through blood infected with HIV. However, since 1985, all donated blood in the United States has been tested for HIV. Therefore, the risk for HIV infection through the transfusion of blood or blood products is extremely low. The U.S. blood supply is considered among the safest in the world.

## THE RISK FACTORS

You may be at increased risk for infection if you have:

- injected drugs or steroids, during which equipment (such as needles, syringes, cotton, water) and blood were shared with others
- had unprotected vaginal, anal, or oral sex (that is, sex without using condoms) with men who have sex with men, multiple partners, or anonymous partners
- exchanged sex for drugs or money
- been given a diagnosis of, or been treated for, hepatitis, tuberculosis (TB), or a sexually transmitted disease (STD) such as syphilis
- received a blood transfusion or clotting factor during 1978-1985
- had unprotected sex with someone who has any of the risk factors listed above

## METHODS OF PREVENTION

Your risk of getting HIV or passing it to someone else depends on several things. Do you know what they are? You might want to talk to someone who knows about HIV. You can also do the following:

- Abstain from sex (do not have oral, anal, or vaginal sex) until you are in a relationship with only one person, are having sex with only each other, and each of you knows the other's HIV status.
    - If both you and your partner have HIV, use condoms to prevent other STDs and possible infection with a different strain of HIV.
    - If only one of you has HIV, use a latex condom and lubricant every time you have sex.
- If you have, or plan to have, more than one sex partner, consider the following:
    - Get tested for HIV

If you are a man who has had sex with other men, get tested at least once a year.

If you are a woman who is planning to get pregnant or who is pregnant, get tested as soon as possible, before you have your baby.

- o Talk about HIV and other STDs with each partner before you have sex.
- o Learn as much as you can about each partner's past behavior (sex and drug use) and consider the risks to your health before you have sex.
- o Ask your partners if they have recently been tested for HIV; encourage those who have not been tested to do so.
- o Use a latex condom and lubricant every time you have sex.
- o If you think you may have been exposed to another STD such as gonorrhea, syphilis, or Chlamydia trachomatis infection, get treatment. These diseases can increase your risk of getting HIV.

- Even if you think you have low risk for HIV infection, get tested whenever you have a regular medical check-up.
- Do not inject illicit drugs (drugs not prescribed by your doctor). You can get HIV through needles, syringes, and other works if they are contaminated with the blood of someone who has HIV. Drugs also cloud your mind, which may result in riskier sex.
- If you do inject drugs, do the following:
  - o Use only clean needles, syringes, and other works.
  - o Never share needles, syringes, or other works.
  - o Be careful not to expose yourself to another person's blood.
  - o Get tested for HIV test at least once a year.
  - o Consider getting counseling and treatment for your drug use.

- Do not have sex when you are taking drugs or drinking alcohol because being high can make you more likely to take risks.

  To protect yourself, remember these ABCs:

  A = Abstinence; B = Be Faithful; C = Condoms.

## SYMPTOMS OF INFECTION

The only way to know whether you are infected is to be tested for HIV. You cannot rely on symptoms alone because many people who are infected with HIV do not have symptoms for many years. Someone can look and feel healthy but can still be infected. In fact, one quarter of the HIV-infected persons in the United States do not know that they are infected.

## HIV TESTING

Once HIV enters the body, the body starts to produce antibodies-substances the immune system creates after infection. Most HIV tests look for these antibodies rather than the virus itself. There are many different kinds of HIV tests, including rapid tests and home test kits. All HIV tests approved by the US government are very good at finding HIV.

## FINDING A TESTING SITE

Many places offer HIV testing: health departments, doctors' offices, hospitals, and sites specifically set up to provide HIV testing.

You can locate a testing site by visiting the CDC HIV testing database or by calling CDC-INFO (formerly the CDC National AIDS Hotline) at 1-800-CDC-INFO (1-800-232-4636) 24 Hours/Day. You do not have to give any personal information about yourself to use these services to find a testing site.

## GRANTS

### General Information

The Centers For Disease Control and Prevention awards grants and cooperative agreements to eligible organizations annually, based on funding made available through its appropriations. All federally funded grants and cooperative agreements are created to provide assistance to accomplish a public purpose. CDC is legislatively mandated to fund only organizations. The funding opportunities at CDC for which interested organizations may apply are designed by the Centers and Offices to carry out the CDC mission of health promotion and preparedness.

Most awards are made through a competitive process. Awards made to one organization only have been designated either by Congress or CDC to be best resource for the public service activity.

The competitive process begins with the publication of the funding opportunity CDC publishes on its website and on grants.gov. This document describes in full detail, the purpose of the award, the requirements for eligibility, estimated award amounts, application timelines and the method of selection. A new funding opportunity announcement will be posted for a period of no less than thirty days.

Following the closing date of the publication, applications will be screened for eligibility. Applications from eligible applicants will be reviewed and scored. Applications for awards that support research are reviewed through a two tier process.The first review is for scientific merit. The second is for programmatic conformance.

Awards are made according to rank score, additional published criteria, if any, and the availability of funds. After all selections have been made, organizations whose applications were reviewed but not funded, will be notified of their status. An application will remain active for one year from the date of notification.

The term men who have sex with men (MSM) refers to all men who have sex with other men, regardless of how they identify themselves (gay, bisexual, or heterosexual). In the United States, HIV and AIDS have had a tremendous impact on MSM. Consider these facts:

- AIDS has been diagnosed for more than half a million MSM. Almost 300,000 MSM with AIDS have died during the past 20 years.

- MSM made up about two thirds of all men living with HIV in 2004, even though only about 5% to 7% of men in the United States reported having sex with other men.
- In a 2005 study, 46% of African American MSM were HIV-positive.

Since HIV/AIDS in MSM was first diagnosed 1981, gay and bisexual men have been leaders in dealing with the challenges of the epidemic. Gay organizations and activists, through their work, have contributed greatly to many of the guidelines for prevention, treatment, and the care of people living with HIV/AIDS.

For complex reasons, HIV/AIDS continues to take a high toll on the MSM population. For example, the number of new HIV/AIDS cases among MSM in 2004 was 8% more than the number of cases in 2003. It is unclear whether this increase is due to more testing or to an increase in the number of HIV infections. Whatever the reasons, in 2004, MSM still accounted for about 51% of all new HIV/AIDS cases and 70% of cases in male adults and adolescents

## An Overview

The Antiretroviral Treatment Access Study II (ARTAS II) demonstration project addresses strategy 3 of the Advancing HIV Prevention (AHP) initiative: prevent new infections by working with HIV-infected persons and their partners. ARTAS II explores the effect of linkage case management on getting HIV-positive persons into care. In the linkage case management approach, a person who has recently received an HIV diagnosis is assigned a linkage case manager to ensure that he or she accesses HIV primary care.

Despite significant successes in preventing and treating HIV infection, the annual estimated number of new HIV infections in the United States has remained at 40,000 for nearly 10 years. A contributor to the steady rate of HIV transmission is the delay between receiving an HIV diagnosis and seeking HIV primary care. After testing positive for HIV, approximately 40% of those receiving this diagnosis delay a year or more before entering primary care.

When people delay entry into care, they do not get the personal and public health benefits of treatment, such as reduced viral load, which can reduce the risk of transmitting HIV. In addition, they miss the counseling that could help reduce their risk for spreading HIV to sex-and needle-sharing partners. As CDC and local health authorities focus on increasing the number of at-risk persons tested for HIV, it is vital that those who test positive for HIV are effectively and rapidly linked to an HIV primary care provider and to ongoing case management when available.

ARTAS II is based on the recently completed ARTAS study. ARTAS showed that when persons with a recent diagnosis of HIV infection meet up to 5 times in a 3-month period with a linkage case manager, they have a greater chance of being linked to care (measured by 2 or more visits to an HIV care provider within a 12-month period). By comparison, persons with a recent diagnosis of HIV infection who receive only a passive referral are less likely to be linked to care. In fact, ARTAS showed that 78% of HIV-infected persons who met with a linkage case manager had stayed in care 6 months later (versus 60% of those who received a passive referral) and that 65% of those who met with a linkage case manager had stayed in care 12 months later (versus 49% of those who received a passive referral).

The ARTAS II demonstration project will compare rates of linkage to HIV care providers before and after instituting the linkage case management shown effective in the first ARTAS study. Findings of the study will strengthen our understanding of how well linkage case management works in typical HIV program settings in the United States.

The 10 collaborating sites for ARTAS II include 5 local or state health departments and 5 community-based organizations (CBOs). Each site will have at least one ARTAS II linkage case manager.

**Goals**

The primary objective of this demonstration project is to achieve a rate of use of HIV care associated with linkage case management of at least 75% after 6 months of follow-up.

The secondary goals of this project are to:

- Determine if the rate achieved during linkage case management is higher than the rate that existed in the community before the ARTAS case management intervention.
- Evaluate the public health impact, based on cost increases or cost savings from the project, on local HIV health care providers and local agencies responsible for HIV diagnosis and case management.
- Explain why there are differences in linkage to HIV care outcome rates across sites.

**Collaborator Projects**

Atlanta, Georgia, AIDS Survival Project is a CBO founded in 1987 by a small group of people living with HIV who wanted to promote self-empowerment and enhanced quality of life for HIV-infected persons. The CBO now provides the Atlanta area with HIV/AIDS education, support services, peer counseling, and, more recently, HIV counseling and testing. It will collaborate with another Atlanta CBO, Our Common Welfare, to provide ARTAS II linkage case management services.

Chicago, Illinois, Alliance for Community Empowerment is a CBO that specializes in HIV/AIDS care and, since 1991, has provided services to clients who are primarily poor, African American, and living on Chicago's South Side. This area is highly impacted by HIV and other public health problems. The alliance will work closely with the HIV Care Center at Michael Reese Hospital to provide linkage case management services to clients.

Jacksonville, Florida, Duval County/Florida Department of Health has provided HIV early intervention services and primary case management since 1986 to residents of Duval Country, Florida. The health department has numerous anonymous and confidential counseling and testing centers within the county, as well as HIV prevention and primary care centers. It serves 60% of the persons diagnosed with HIV infection or AIDS in Duval County. Staff members intend to incorporate ARTAS II linkage case management into their existing care services. Anniston, Alabama, Health Services Center, Inc. (HSC) is a one-stop shop for HIV/AIDS care in rural northeast Alabama. Since the original clinic was founded in 1987, it has expanded its services to include primary medical care, case management, outreach and retention, adherence, palliative care programs, HIV prevention, and mental health and substance abuse treatment and prevention activities. HSC plans for ARTAS II linkage case managers to work closely with disease intervention specialists to link persons with new HIV diagnoses to medical care.

Kansas City, Missouri, Kansas City Free Health Clinic is a free, volunteer-driven clinic that provides over 25,000 patient encounters annually in general medicine, mental health, dental, and HIV primary care. Started in 1971 to serve underserved youth, it has become the largest provider of HIV primary care, prevention, and outreach in Greater Kansas City (both Kansas and Missouri). It is also a publicly funded HIV testing site, offering the only anonymous testing in the area. The clinic expects to use ARTAS II funding to develop a formal system to track client engagement from testing to retention in care.

New Orleans, Louisiana, Louisiana Department of Health and Hospitals oversees the state's HIV prevention, services, and surveillance programs. The health department intends to collaborate with two experienced CBOs-Family Service of Greater Baton Rouge and Volunteers of America-to provide linkage case management services to persons living with HIV/AIDS in the greater Baton Rouge/Region II area. Region II is largely rural, but the city of Baton Rouge ranks second in the nation in AIDS case rates among large cities.

Miami, Florida, Miami-Dade County/Florida Department of Health maintains, in collaboration with the University of Miami School of Medicine, three clinics (downtown Miami, South Beach, and South Dade County) dedicated to sexually transmitted disease and HIV counseling and testing. Their staffs intend to recruit participants from these clinics for the project. They also intend to collaborate with the South Florida AIDS Network, the largest CBO in Miami, to provide medical care to persons living with HIV. The Miami-Dade County Health Department collaborated with the University of Miami on the initial ARTAS clinical trial. Columbia, South Carolina, South Carolina Department of Health and Environmental Control plans to implement ARTAS II in two metropolitan areas-Columbia and Greenville-which together account for about 309 new HIV cases annually. It plans to recruit project participants primarily through local health department HIV counseling and testing services and collaborate with two CBOs (Midlands Care Consortia and AID Upstate) to provide linkage case management.

Baltimore, Maryland, Total Health Care, Inc. has provided primary health care to the poor and medically underserved residents of Baltimore City since 1989. It has five sites, and the area it serves accounts for over 80% of all newly diagnosed HIV cases in the city. It is one of only four organizations in Baltimore that provide HIV counseling and testing, case management, and primary care. ARTAS II funds will be used to help link persons recently diagnosed with HIV to HIV medical care as soon as possible after diagnosis.

Richmond, Virginia, Virginia Department of Health intends to contract with Virginia Commonwealth University (VCU) and its entities, the Central Virginia HIV CARE Consortium (CVHCC) and the Surgery and Evaluation Research Laboratory (SERL) to implement ARTAS II. VCU will coordinate its linkage case management services with publicly funded counseling and testing sites and with HIV care providers in CVHCC and SERL.

**Project Milestones**

- Funding announcement: June 2004
- Grant recipients announced: September 2004
- Grantee orientation meeting: November 2004
- Grantees attend strengths-based case management training in Dayton, OH: January 2005
- Grantees attend data manager training in Atlanta, GA: March 2005
- Client enrollment begins: April 2005
- 6-month follow-up begins: October 2005
- 12-month follow-up begins: May 2006

## Data Collection

Data measuring program effectiveness will be collected through 1-on-1 interviews with clients, A—CASI (audio-computer assisted self-interviewing), and medical records abstraction to verify client self-report.

Pre-intervention data will be collected from state HIV/AIDS reporting and Ryan White and Medicaid encounter data to establish a baseline rate of linkage to HIV care. These data will include date of positive confirmatory HIV test, HIV exposure category or categories, race, ethnicity, and, in some cases, date of HIV care encounter. Data collected through the ARTAS II demonstration project will be primarily sociodemographic data, although some questions will elicit data on HIV testing, drug use, risk behaviors, depression, and knowledge, attitudes, and beliefs about HIV/AIDS.

At 6 and 12 months after an initial case management visit, each client will be contacted by the project site to return for a follow-up A-CASI to determine if he or she has had medical care since joining the study. The follow-up interviews contain additional questions that elicit data on select barriers to engaging in HIV primary care. The client's medical record will also be abstracted at that time to verify client self-report.

Program evaluation will measure any increase in the percentage of clients linked to medical care within 12 months of their HIV diagnosis compared with the pre-intervention population. The effect of ongoing case management on linkage to medical care will also be evaluated by comparing rates of linkage to care among those clients who become linked to ongoing case management with rates among those who do not.

## Results to Date

As of June 2006:

- Data collection is in progress and will continue through January 2007 for all 10 sites.
- Enrollment is still in progress for 3 grantee sites.
- 609 clients have been enrolled and have completed the baseline ACASI survey.

- 198 clients have completed the 6-month ACASI survey.
- 43 clients have completed the 12-month ACASI survey.
- Medical record abstractions are in progress.
- Data collection to assess client, agency level, and case manger level program costs is ongoing.
- Pre-intervention linkage rate data collection is ongoing.
- Site visits to all 10 grantees have been completed.
- Preliminary estimates of program cost for the case management intervention have been calculated.

Incorporating HIV Prevention into Medical Care Settings (PICS) demonstration project addresses strategies 1 and 3 of the Advancing HIV Prevention Initiative. It will explore the effects of clinic-based, repeated, brief prevention counseling on patient behaviors and sexually transmitted diseases (STDs) in the United States through a program called Positive S.T.E.P.s (Striving to Engage People).

After testing positive for HIV, many people reduce behaviors that may transmit HIV to others; however, such behavioral changes are not always maintained and some people continue to engage in behaviors that place themselves and others at risk. Ongoing, brief prevention counseling is a cost-effective measure that can be incorporated into routine care for HIV-positive individuals. The HIV outpatient clinic is an ideal setting for the delivery of this intervention to large numbers of individuals with HIV in the years following their HIV diagnosis because it provides an opportunity to a) reach a large number of seropositive individuals who visit the clinic on a regular basis, b) implement a safer-sex and needle-sharing intervention across time, c) integrate the intervention with routine clinical care, and d) involve clinic nurses and physicians in the intervention.

The six sites chosen for this project implemented the 2003 Incorporating HIV Prevention into Medical Care Settings Guidelines and assessed their impact on patient-reported risk behaviors, STD rates, tailored risk-reduction counseling, and referrals. Providers at participating sites received training to enhance their HIV prevention and risk-reduction planning and counseling skills. Mountain Plains AIDS Education Training

Center (MPAETC) was contracted to provide standardized training at each of the six clinics, as well as a variety of prevention posters and brochures geared toward patients and providers.

**Goals**

The goals of this program are to:

- recruit 1,200 patients at six sites (200 per site) with at least 50% racial/ethnic minority representation,
- increase the number of persons with HIV who have information about transmission risks and regularly receive counseling about ways to reduce the risk of transmitting HIV to others,
- increase the number of sexually active persons with HIV who are screened and tested for STDs,
- enhance the capacity and ability to conduct effective prevention counseling and referral for services (e.g., social, mental health, drug treatment, partner notification), and
- assist in strengthening linkages among health departments, CBOs, and providers of HIV care to facilitate the referral of HIV-positive persons to needed services.

# 3

# HIV/AIDS: The Indian Scenario

India has among the highest number of persons living with HIV/AIDS in the world today, although the overall prevalence remains low. Some states experience a generalized epidemic with the virus transmitted from high-risk groups into the general population. A major challenge is to strengthen and decentralize the program to the state and district levels to enhance commitment, coverage and effectiveness.

## STATE OF THE EPIDEMIC

There are more than 5.1 million individuals infected with HIV in this country of over 1 billion people (UNAIDS 2003). The total number of AIDS cases in 2002 was estimated to be about 550,000. Seven states-Andhra Pradesh, Goa, Karnataka, Maharashtra, Manipur, Mizoram, and Nagaland-already have generalized epidemics, as indicated by a 1 percent or higher prevalence rate among pregnant women in prenatal clinics. These seven states represent 22 percent of the population.

## RISK AND VULNERABILITY

Several factors put India in danger of experiencing a rapid spread if effective prevention and control measures are not scaled up and expanded throughout the country. These risk factors include:Unsafe Sex and Low Condom Use: In India, sexual transmission is responsible for 84 percent of reported AIDS cases. HIV-prevalence rates are highest among sex workers and their clients, injecting drug users, and men who have sex with men (many of whom are married). When surveyed, 70 percent of commercial sex workers in India reported that their main reason for not using of condoms was because their customers objected. Migration and Mobility: Migration for work for extended periods of time takes migrants away from the social environment provided by their families and community. This can place them outside the usual normative constraints and thus more likely to engage in risky behavior. Concerted efforts are needed to address the vulnerabilities of the large migrant population.

## INJECTING DRUG USE (IDU)

Studies indicate that many drug users are switching from inhaling to injecting drugs. This phenomenon is more localized in the Northeastern states of India, and injecting drug users show sharp increases in HIV prevalence. Forty-one percent of IDUs in a national survey reported injecting with used needles or syringes. Of those who cleaned their needles and syringes, only three percent used an effective method such as alcohol, bleach, or boiling water. Appropriate strategies are also needed to address the double impact of drug use and unsafe sexual practices.

## LOW STATUS OF WOMEN

Infection rates have been on the increase among women and infants in some states. As in many other countries, unequal power relations and the low status of women, as expressed by limited access to human, financial, and economic assets, weakens the ability of women to protect themselves and negotiate safer sex, thereby increasing vulnerability.

## WIDESPREAD STIGMA

Stigma towards people infected with HIV/AIDS is widespread. The misconception that AIDS only affects men who have sex with men, sex workers, and injecting drug users strengthens and perpetuates existing discrimination. The most affected groups, often marginalized, have little or no access to legal protection of their basic human rights. Addressing the issue of human rights violations and creating an enabling environment that increases knowledge and encourages behavior change are thus extremely important to the fight against AIDS.

## National Response to HIV/AIDS

**Government:** Shortly after reporting the first AIDS case in 1986, the Government of India established a National AIDS Control Program (NACP) which was managed by a small unit within the Ministry of Health and Family Welfare. The program's principal activity was then limited to monitoring HIV infection rates among risk populations in select urban areas. In 1991, the strategy was revised to focus on blood safety, prevention among high-risk populations, raising awareness in the general population, and improving surveillance. A semi-autonomous body, the National AIDS Control Organization (NACO), was established under the Ministry of Health and Family Welfare to implement this program. This "first phase" of the National AIDS Control Program lasted from 1992-1999. It focused on initiating a national commitment, increasing awareness and addressing blood safety. It achieved some of its objectives, notably an increased awareness.

Professional blood donations were banned by law. Screening of donated blood became almost universal by the end of this phase. However, performance across states remained variable. By 1999, the program had also established a decentralized mechanism to facilitate effective state-level responses, although substantial variation continued to exist in the level of commitment and capacity among states. Whereas states such as Tamil Nadu, Andhra Pradesh, and Manipur demonstrated a strong response and high level of political commitment, many other states, such as Bihar and Uttar Pradesh, have yet to reach these levels. The second phase of the NACP began in 1999 and will run until March 2006. Under this phase, India continues to expand the program at the state level. Greater emphasis has been placed on targeted interventions for high-risk groups, preventive interventions among the general population, and involvement of NGOs and other sectors and line departments, such as education, transport and police.

Capacity and accountability at the state level continues to be a major issue and has required sustained support. Interventions need to be scaled up to cover a higher percentage of the population, and monitoring and evaluation need further strengthening. The Government has done away with the classification of states based on prevalence to avoid inducing complacency among states categorized as low prevalence, and has since focused on the vulnerability of states, hence creating a sense of urgency. In brief, while the government's response has scaled up markedly over the last decade, major challenges remain in raising the overall effectiveness of state-level programs, expanding the participation of other sectors, and increasing safe behavior and reducing stigma associated with HIV-positive people among the population. The Government of India is currently in the early stages of preparing for the third phase of the National AIDS Control Program (NACP 3), for which a multi-disciplinary design team has been constituted to lead the preparation. The design of NACP 3 envisages a complex consultative process including nationwide consultations with various national stakeholders, as well as international development partners.

## NON-GOVERNMENTAL ORGANIZATIONS (NGOs)

There are numerous NGOs working on HIV/AIDS issues in India at the local, state, and national levels. Projects include targeted interventions with high risk groups; direct care of people living with HIV/AIDS; general awareness campaigns; and care for AIDS orphans. Funding for NGOs comes from a variety of sources: the federal or state governments of India, international donors, and local contributions. Donors: India receives technical assistance and funding from a variety of UN partners and bilateral donors. Bilateral donors such as USAID, CIDA, and DFID have been involved since the early 1990s at the state level in a number of states. USAID has committed more than US$70 million since 1992, CIDA US$11 million, and DFID close to US$200 million.

The number of major financers and the amount of funding available has increased significantly in the last year. Since 2004, the Gates Foundation has pledged US$200 million for the next five years, the Global Fund has approved US$26 million for Prevention of Mother-to-Child Transmission (PMTCT) and about US$7 million for TB/HIV co-infection, and is considering another round of proposals, and USAID is considering the inclusion of India as its 15th priority country.

DFID has also increased its financing and is considering the inclusion of additional states. Other more recent donors include DANIDA, SIDA, the Clinton Foundation and the European Union.

## ISSUES AND CHALLENGES

### Priority Areas

Limited Overall Capacity: There are severe institutional capacity constraints, including managerial, at the national and state levels. These are critical factors to address as the program attempts to scale-up the national response. NACO will require a change in its role and responsibilities to provide the necessary leadership and steering role for a stronger multisector response for the next phase in India's fight against HIV/AIDS.

### Variable Ability to Implement Responses Across States

The capacity to mount a strong program is weakest in some of the poorest and most populated states with significant vulnerability to the epidemic. There is a need for tailored capacity-building activities and the introduction of some performance-based financing approaches. Institutional arrangements and personnel turnover: There is a high turnover of state level project directors, resulting in limited continuity and variability in performance across states. This puts program growth at risk.

### Donor Coordination

At present there are over 32 donor agencies working with NACO in different states and on different programs. Each donor comes with its own mandate and requirements, as well as areas of focus. The transaction cost to the government as a result of attending to the various demands of the donors is huge. There is a need for better coordinating mechanisms among the donors and clear leadership by the Government to reduce the transaction costs.

### Use of Data for Decision Making

There remains a need for greater use of data for decision making, including program data and epidemiological data. A lot of data that is being generated is not adequately used for managing the program or inform policies and priorities. Results-based management and linking incentives to the use of data should be explored. Stigma and Discrimination: Stigma and discrimination against people living with HIV/AIDS and those considered to be at high risk remain entrenched. A lot of this is a result of inadequate knowledge. For instance, more than 75 percent of Indians mistakenly believed they could contract HIV from sharing a meal with a person who has the disease, according to a recent study. Stigma and denial undermine efforts to increase the coverage of effective interventions among high risk groups such as men having sex with men, commercial sex workers and injecting drug users. Harassment by police and ostracism by family and community drives the epidemic underground and decreases the reach and effectiveness of prevention efforts. Though there is significant increase in awareness, due to efforts by the government, there is much room for improvement.

### Low Awareness in Rural Areas

Sentinel site behavioral surveillance, completed in 2001, showed high HIV/AIDS basic awareness levels (82.4 percent in males and 70 percent in females). However, rural women demonstrated very low rates of awareness in Bihar (21.5 percent), Gujarat (25 percent), and Uttar Pradesh (27.6 percent). New approaches need to be tried to reach rural communities with information about HIV/AIDS, safe sex and how to prevent and treat HIV/AIDS.

## WORLD BANK RESPONSE

In 1991, the Government of India and the World Bank expanded their collaboration on infectious disease control programs and by 1992 the first National AIDS Control Project was launched with a World Bank credit of US$84 million. The project helped the government to broaden prevention efforts and to establish institutions and procedures necessary to curb the spread of HIV/AIDS. Building upon lessons learned from the first project, India requested World Bank financing for a follow-on project. With a World Bank credit of US$191 million, the Second National HIV/AIDS Control Project was started and this is increasing the pace of implementation through the use of State AIDS Societies to speed the distribution of funds at the state level.

The Bank has also undertaken analytical work to strengthen the national response, including an analysis of the full array of costs and consequences likely to result from several plausible government policy options regarding funding for anti-retroviral therapy (ART). Currently, the Bank is carrying out sector work on the economic consequences of the HIV/AIDS epidemic on India and is actively supporting the design of the third National AIDS Control Program.

## CONTROLLING TECHNIQUES

Controlling HIV/AIDS in India is an "immense" challenge for the country's National AIDS Control Organization—which is preparing to launch on April 1 the third phase of its National AIDS Control Program, a new five-year, $2.6 billion program that aims to reduce the number of new HIV cases and improve access to treatment in the country.

NEJM national correspondent Robert Steinbrook writes in a perspective piece. According to Steinbrook, two-thirds of NACP-III program's budget will go toward prevention efforts, while one-sixth will go toward providing treatment access to HIV-positive people. He adds that although prevention efforts will "account for a smaller percentage of the total NACP resources than at present," prevention "will remain the focus of India's AIDS control strategy." Steinbrook writes that the challenges associated with providing treatment access and preventing the spread of HIV in India include "increasing the number of patients receiving treatment, making additional medications available, improving the monitoring of therapy, training physicians and other health care workers, caring for patients with tuberculosis coinfection, and reducing stigma and discrimination." Steinbrook adds that NACP's "immediate priorities" are "to start patients on first-line regimens, to achieve high rates of compliance through supervised therapy and intensive counseling, to build infrastructure," and—according to NACO Director-General Sujatha Rao—to ensure that people are not "dying for lack of access to drugs that are available and affordable." Steinbrook concludes that the "new phase of the AIDS control program is just beginning, and the challenges remain immense".

Providing access to care to people living with HIV/TB coinfection also is a "major public health challenge" in India, Steinbrook writes in a second NEJM perspective piece. According to Steinbrook, people with HIV/TB coinfection have "higher risks of recurrence and death," and TB is "expected to develop in more than half" of HIV-positive people in India. Treatments for TB and HIV are "increasingly being coordinated, but the full benefits have yet to be realized," Steinbrook writes. Steinbrook concludes that the "control of both [TB] and HIV is likely to be most successful if programs collaborate whenever possible and are closely integrated with the rest of medical care" India has had a sharp increase in the estimated number of HIV infections, from the first reported case in 1986 in chennai among a commercial sex worker, then escalating to several thousand in the early 1990s to around five million in 2003. National estimates have come under scrutiny and are generally considered to be underestimations of the true absolute number of persons living with HIV in India.

India's national epidemic is made up of a number of local epidemics, and in some places they occur within the same state. The epidemics vary, from states with mainly heterosexual transmission of HIV, often via interaction with sex workers, to some states where intravenous drug use is the main route of transmission. Both tracking the epidemic and implementing effective programmes poses a serious challenge to the authorities and communities in India. HIV surveillance in India falls under the auspices of the National AIDS Control Organization (NACO). The majority of HIV surveillance data collected by NACO is done through annual unlinked anonymous testing of prenatal clinic (or antenatal clinics) and sexually transmitted infection clinic attendees.

India has a large population and population density, low literacy levels and consequently low levels of awareness, and HIV/AIDS is one of the most challenging public health problems ever faced by the country. A recent study published in the British medical journal "The Lancet" in (2006) reported an approximately 30% decline in HIV infections among young women aged 15 to 24 years attending prenatal clinics in selected southern states of India from 2000 to 2004 where the epidemic is thought to be concentrated. The authors cautiously attribute observed declines to increased condom use by men who visit commercial sex workers and cite several pieces of corroborating evidence. Acquired Immune Deficiency Syndrome (AIDS) has killed more than 25 million people since it was first recognized in 1981, making it one of the most destructive epidemics in recorded history. Despite recent improved access to antiretroviral treatment and care in many regions of the world, the AIDS epidemic claimed approximately 3.1 million (between 2.8 and 3.6 million) lives in 2005 (an average of 8,500 per day), of which 570,000 were children.

UNAIDS and the WHO estimate that the total number of people living with the human immunodeficiency virus (HIV) has reached its highest level. There are an estimated 40.3 million (estimated range between 36.7 and 45.3 million) people now living with HIV. Moreover, almost 5 million people have been estimated to have been infected with HIV in 2005 alone.

The epidemic is not homogeneous within regions with some countries more afflicted than others. Even at the country level there are wide variations in infection levels between different areas. The number of people living with HIV continues to rise in most parts of the world, despite strenuous prevention strategies. Sub-Saharan Africa remains by far the worst-affected region, with 23.8 million to 28.9 million people living with HIV at the end of 2005, 1 million more than in 2003. Sixty-four percent of all people living with HIV are in sub-Saharan Africa, as are more than 77% of all women living with HIV. South & South East Asia are second most affected with 15%.

The key facts surrounding this origin of AIDS are currently unknown, particularly where and when the pandemic began, though it is said that it originated from the apes in Africa.

## ORIGIN AND SPREAD OF AIDS

AIDS is thought to have originated in sub-Saharan Africa during the 20th century. It was transferred to humans by a similar route as some classic Old World infectious diseases. The ancient Old World was the incubator of many diseases like smallpox because it had large human populations in close association with large animal populations, especially those that lived in herds or social groups.

## Possible Spread from Animal to Human Populations

HIV originated in non-human primates as far as is known. Researchers announced in May 2006 that the HIV virus most likely originated in wild chimpanzees in the southeastern rain forests of Cameroon (modern East Province) rather than in Kinshasa, Democratic Republic of Congo (formerly Zaire), as had previously been believed. Seven years of research and 1,300 chimpanzee genetic samples led Dr. Beatrice Hahn of the University of Alabama, Birmingham, to identify chimpanzee communities near Cameroon's Sanaga River as the most likely originators. The researchers say that transference from chimp to human most likely occurred when a human was bitten by a chimp or was cut while butchering one, and the human became infected. Calculating based on a fixed mutation rate, the jump from chimpanzee to human likely occurred during the French colonial period (1919-1960). Comparative primatologist Jim Moore suggests that this may have been the result of colonial practices of forced labour, which could have suppressed the immune system of the initial hunter enough to allow the virus to infect and take hold. Likewise, forced immunisations (using one needle on many patients) may have sped the virus's spread through Cameroon and beyond.

A more controversial theory known as the OPV AIDS hypothesis suggests that the AIDS epidemic was inadvertently started in the Belgian Congo by Hilary Koprowski's 1950s research into a polio vaccine prepared from tissue cultures using locally captured non-human primates. Edward Hooper rejects the dates calculated using a fixed mutation rate on the basis that phylogenetic dating of "the most recombinogenic organisms known to medical science", immunodeficiency viruses, is "inherently incapable of making any allowance for recombination". However, in February 2000 one of the original developers of the polio vaccine, Philadelphia based Wistar Institute found in its stores a phial of the original vaccine used in the vaccination program. It was analysed in April 2001 and no traces of either HIV-1 or SIV were found in the sample. A second analysis showed that only macaque monkey kindney cells, which cannot be infected with SIV or HIV, were used to produce the vaccine. While the analysis was done on only one phial of vaccine, most scientists have concluded that the polio vaccine theory of the origins of HIV is not possible.

After the initial transfer of HIV from a non-human primate to humans, the virus ultimately spread via contact among humans to the rest of the world. Since a cross species jump is most likely the origin of HIV, and since HIV became a true epidemic, transmissible from human to human, then the following conditions were needed:

1. A large human population,
2. A large nearby population of the appropriate host animal,
3. An infectious pathogen in the host animal, that eventually produces a mutation that can spread from animal to human,
4. Interaction between the species to transmit enough of it to humans to establish a human foothold, which may take millions of individual exposures,
5. A mutation of same pathogen that can spread from human to human,
6. Some method that allows the pathogen to disperse widely. This prevents the infection from "burning out" by either killing off its human hosts or provoking immunity in a local population of humans.

Such requirements existed in the remote past with smallpox, and also with the 20th century Spanish Flu, despite the latter's New World origin at Fort Riley, Kansas (there the animal reservoir seems to have been two species, chickens and pigs, which were of Old World origin.)

Two species of HIV infect humans: HIV-1 and HIV-2. HIV-1 is more virulent and more easily transmitted. HIV-1 is the source of the majority of HIV infections throughout the world, while HIV-2 is less easily transmitted and is largely confined to West Africa.

Both species of the virus (HIV-1 and HIV-2) are believed to have originated in West-Central Africa and jumped species (zoonosis) from a non-human primate to humans. HIV-1 evolved from a Simian Immunodeficiency Virus (SIVcpz) found in the chimpanzee subspecies Pan troglodytes DNA sequencing indicates that HIV-1 (group M) entered the human population in the early 20th century, probably sometime between 1915 and 1941. HIV-2 crossed species from a different strain of SIV, this one found in sooty mangabeys (an Old World monkey) of Guinea-Bissau.

SIVs in non-human primates tend to cause non-fatal disease. Comparison of the gene sequence of SIV with HIV should therefore give us information about the factors necessary to cause disease in humans. The factors that determine the virulence of HIV as compared to most SIVs are only now being elucidated. Non-human SIVs contain a nef gene that down-regulates CD3, CD4, and MHC class I expression; most non-human SIV's therefore do not induce immunodeficiency; the HIV nef gene however has lost its ability to down-regulate CD3, which results in the immune activation and apoptosis that is characteristic of chronic HIV infection.

## HISTORY OF KNOWN CASES

One of the earliest documented HIV-1 infection dates from 1959, and was discovered in the preserved blood sample of a man from Leopoldville, Belgian Congo (now Kinshasa, Democratic Republic of the Congo). However, it is unknown whether this anonymous person ever developed AIDS and died of its complications. The oldest documented case of the then-unknown syndrome was detected that same year, when a 25-year-old British sailor who had traveled in the navy between 1955 and 1957 (but apparently not to Africa), sought help at the Royal Infirmary of Manchester, England. He reported to have been suffering from puzzling symptoms, among them purplish skin lesions, for nearly two years. His condition had taken a turn for worse during Christmas 1958, when he started suffering from shortness of breath, extreme fatigue, rapid weight loss, night sweats and high fever. The doctors thought he might be suffering from tuberculosis and, even though they found no evidence of bacterial infection, they treated him for tuberculosis just to be safe, to no avail.

The sailor continued to weaken and he died shortly after in August 1959. His autopsy revealed evidence of two unusual infections, cytomegalovirus and Pneumocystis carinii pneumonia (PCP, later, when redetermined as P. jirovecii, renamed Pneumocystis pneumonia) very rare at the time but now commonly associated with AIDS patients. His case had puzzled his doctors, who preserved tissue samples from him and for years retained some interest in solving the mystery. Sir Robert Platt, then president of the Royal College of Physicians, wrote in the sailor's hospital chart that he wondered "if we are in for a new wave of virus disease now that the bacterial illnesses are so nearly conquered". It was only 31 years later, after the AIDS pandemic had become well-known and widespread, that they decided to perform HIV-tests on the preserved tissues of the sailor, which eventually turned out a positive result. The case was reported in the July 7, 1990 issue of the British medical journal The Lancet; their claim was retracted in a letter in the January 20, 1996 issue where they admitted that the tissue sample was contaminated in the laboratory. Another early case was probably detected that same year, 1959, in a 48-year-old Haitian, who 30 years before had immigrated to the United States and at the time was working as a shipping clerk for a garment manufacturer in Manhattan. He developed similar symptoms to those just described for the British sailor, and died the same year, apparently of the same very rare kind of pneumonia. Many years later, Dr. Gordon R. Hennigar, who had performed this man's autopsy, was asked whether he thought his patient had died of AIDS; he replied "You bet" and added "It was so unusual at the time. Lord knows how many cases of AIDS have been autopsied that we didn't even know had AIDS. I think it's such a strong possibility that I've often thought about getting them to send me the tissue samples."

In 1969, a 15-year-old African-American male died at the St. Louis City Hospital from aggressive Kaposi's sarcoma. AIDS was suspected as early as 1984, and in 1987, researchers at Tulane University School of Medicine confirmed this, finding HIV-1 in his preserved blood and tissues. The doctors who worked on his case at the time suspected he was a prostitute, though the patient did not discuss his sexual history with them in detail.

In 1976, a Norwegian sailor named Arvid Noe, his wife, and his nine-year-old daughter died of AIDS. The sailor had first presented symptoms in 1969, four years after he had spent time in ports along the West African coastline. Tissue samples from the sailor and his wife were tested in 1988 and found to contain the HIV-1 virus (Group O). The next documented western death from AIDS was that of Dr. Grethe Rask in 1977. Rask, a Danish surgeon, had worked in the Congo in the early 1970s.

It thus appears that either HIV existed in very low levels in the United States in periods prior to 1981, or it may have gone extinct in the United States at times, with the present infection established in the USA about 1976. HIV in Africa likewise was at first at levels too low to be noticed. In the United States and Africa HIV was at first mostly found only in residents of large cities. The infection is now more widespread in rural areas, and has appeared in regions such as China and India, where it was previously not evident.

Author Randy Shilts mentioned that what was later called AIDS became evident in the gay community in the Fire Island, New York area in the four years after the 1976 Bicentennial celebrations. The infection tended to double in numbers about every nine to ten months. It therefore took a couple of years before a new disease was suspected because there were at first not enough symptomatic individuals to be noticed.

The official date for the beginning of the AIDS epidemic is marked as June 5, 1981, when the US Centers for Disease Control and Prevention reported in its Morbidity and Mortality Weekly Report newsletter that unusual clusters of Pneumocystis carinii pneumonia had been discovered in gay men in Los Angeles in the early 1980s. Over the next eighteen months, more PCP clusters were discovered among otherwise healthy men in cities throughout the country, along with other opportunistic diseases (such as Kaposi's sarcoma and persistent, generalized lymphadenopathy), common in immunosuppressed patients.

In June 1982, a report of a group of cases amongst gay men in Southern California suggested that a sexually transmitted infectious agent might be the etiological agent, and the syndrome was initially termed 'GRID' (Gay-Related Immune Deficiency). However, the same opportunistic infections also began to be reported among hemophiliacs, heterosexual intravenous drug users, and Haitian immigrants. By August 1982, the disease was being referred to by its new name: Acquired Immune Deficiency Syndrome (AIDS). An anagram of AIDS, SIDA, was then coined for use in Portuguese (Síndrome da Imunodeficiência Adquirida) in French (Syndrome d'Immuno-Déficience Acquise) and Spanish (Síndrome de Inmunodeficiencia Adquirida). In Russian it got the name SPID (Sindrom Priobretyonnoy Immunitetnoy Defitsitnosti)

## IDENTIFICATION OF THE VIRUS

In May 1983, doctors from Dr. Luc Montagnier's team at the Pasteur Institute in France, reported that they had isolated a new retrovirus from lymphoid ganglions that they believed was the cause of AIDS. The virus was later named lymphadenopathy-associated virus (LAV) and a sample was sent to the U.S. Centers for Disease Control, which was later passed to the National Cancer Institute (NCI).

In May 1984, Dr Robert Gallo of the NCI also isolated a virus that caused AIDS, and named it Human T-cell Lymphotropic Virus-III (HTLV-III). In January 1985 a number of more detailed reports were published concerning LAV and HTLV-III, and by March it was clear that the viruses were the same, from the same source, and was the etiological agent of AIDS. In May 1986, the International Committee on the Taxonomy of Viruses ruled that both names should be dropped and a new name, HIV (Human Immunodeficiency Virus), be used.

A United States HIV/AIDS Memorial Museum, to be located in Newark, New Jersey, USA, is being planned. Its first pilot program, an exhibit of art by HIV-positive artists, was held from November 11 through December 1, 2006 at Seton Hall University in South Orange, NJ. The AIDS Museum's second exhibit will be hosted at Seton Hall Law School in Newark, NJ.

**The Mission Statement of the Organization Is:** "The AIDS Museum will be America's national institution for the documentation, study and interpretation of the AIDS pandemic. The mission of the Museum will be to advance and disseminate knowledge about AIDS, to preserve the memory of those who have died and continue to suffer, and to encourage visitors to reflect upon the medical, political, and humanitarian questions raised by the AIDS pandemic. The Museum will have an inspirational tone, highlighting the ways in which people have come together through organizations to creatively address the range of social and health care issues raised by the pandemic."

There is currently an AIDS Museum located in Thailand and another being developed in South Africa.

While there are AIDS memorials, exhibits, and artwork in the United States, the AIDS Museum in Newark will be the first institution of its kind in the country.

# 4

# HIV/AIDS Cases in India

**FAST FACTS**

India is experiencing rapid and extensive spread of HIV. This is particularly worrisome since India is home to a population of over 900 million. As a single nation it has more people than the continents of Africa, Australia and Latin America combined.

- There are an estimated 2 to 5 million people infected with HIV in India today, and 50,000 to 100,000 cases of AIDS may have already occurred in the country.
- This epidemic is fueled by both married and unmarried men visiting sex workers.
- The most rapid and well-documented spread of HIV has occurred in Bombay and the State of Tamil Nadu. In Bombay HIV prevalence has reached the level of 50 percent in sex workers, 36 percent in STD patients and 2.5 percent in women attending antenatal clinics.
- Certain regions, such as eastern India (Calcutta area) and northern India (New Delhi region), still show a lower prevalence of HIV (1 to 2 percent) among sex workers.
- Contrary to traditional belief, sexually transmitted diseases and sex with multiple partners are common in the country, both in urban and rural areas. An estimated 3 to 4 percent of some rural populations have a sexually transmitted disease.
- Injecting drug use is a problem in Manipur, which is in the North East region, where 55 percent of drug users

are HIV-infected and 1 percent of women attending antenatal clinics are infected with HIV.

- HIV is rapidly spreading to rural areas through migrant workers and truck drivers. Surveys show that 5 to 10 percent of some truck drivers in the country are infected with HIV.
- An estimated 1 to 2 million cases of tuberculosis occur in India every year. In Bombay 10 percent of the patients presenting with tuberculosis are HIV-positive. Tuberculosis is the presenting symptom of AIDS in over 60 percent of AIDS cases.
- A major international and governmental effort is necessary to respond effectively to this severe epidemic.

India has a population of one billion, around half of whom are adult-sin the sexually active age group. The first AIDS case in India was detected in 1986, and since then HIV infection has been reported in all States and Union Territories.

The spread of HIV in India has been diverse, with much of India having a low rate of infection and the epidemic being most extreme in the southern half of the country and in the far north-east. The highest HIV prevalence rates are found in Maharashtra in the west; Andhra Pradesh and Karnataka in the south; and Manipur and Nagaland in the north-east.

***Estimated number of people living with HIV/AIDS, end of 2005***

| Group | Living with HIV/AIDS |
|---|---|
| Adults and children | 5,700,000 |
| Adults | 5,600,000 |
| Women | 1,600,000 |
| Adult HIV prevalence estimate | 0.9% |

As of August 2006, 90% of all nationally reported AIDS cases have been found in 10 of the 38 States Union Territories. The greatest numbers were in Maharashtra and Gujarat in the west; Tamil Nadu, Andhra Pradesh and Karnataka in the south; and Manipur and West Bengal in the north-east.

In the southern States, the infections are mostly due to heterosexual contact, while infections are mainly found amongst injecting drug users in Manipur and Nagaland.

These are UNAIDS/WHO estimates. 3 Adults are defined as people aged 15 or above. These estimates include all those with HIV infection, whether or not they have developed symptoms of AIDS.

The Indian National AIDS Control Organization (NACO) estimates that 5.21 million people were living with HIV in 2005, giving an adult prevalence of 0.91%. This represents a slight increase from the 2004 estimate, and a substantial increase from 4.58 million in 2002.

***AIDS data, end of August 2006***

| Gender | Cumulative AIDS Cases |
|---|---|
| Male | 88,245 |
| Female | 36,750 |
| Total | 124,995 |

The statistics for AIDS cases may be a poor guide to the severity of the epidemic, as in many situations a patient will die without HIV having been diagnosed, and with the cause of death attributed to an opportunistic infection, such as tuberculosis.

***According to UNAIDS/WHO, between 270,000 and 680,000 Indians died of AIDS in 2005.***

| Transmission Categories | Number of cases | % |
|---|---|---|
| Sexual | 106,669 | 85% |
| Mother-to-child | 4,755 | 4% |
| Blood and blood products | 2,563 | 2% |
| Injecting drug users | 2,930 | 2% |
| Others (not specified) | 8,078 | 6% |
| Total | 124,995 | 100% |

| Age group | Male | Female | Total |
|---|---|---|---|
| 0-14 | 3,313 | 2,283 | 5,596 |
| 15-29 | 23,905 | 15,876 | 39,781 |
| 30-49 | 54,204 | 16,701 | 70,905 |
| =50 | 6,823 | 1,890 | 8,713 |
| Total | 88,245 | 36,750 | 124,995 |

| State/Union Territory | AIDS cases |
|---|---|
| A & N Islands | 37 |
| Andhra Pradesh | 15,099 |
| Arunachal Pradesh | 13 |
| Assam | 372 |
| Bihar | 155 |
| Chandigarh (UT) | 1,934 |
| Chattisgarh | 0 |
| Daman & Diu | 1 |
| Dadra & Nagar Haveli | 0 |
| Delhi | 2,759 |
| Goa | 657 |
| Gujarat | 6,873 |
| Haryana | 655 |
| Himachal Pradesh | 302 |
| Jammu & Kashmir | 2 |
| Jharkhand | 258 |
| Karnataka | 4,385 |
| Kerala | 1,769 |
| Lakshadweep | 0 |
| Madhya Pradesh | 1,729 |
| Maharashtra | 14,325 |
| Manipur | 2,866 |
| Meghalaya | 8 |

*Contd...*

| State/Union Territory | AIDS cases |
|---|---|
| Mizoram | 106 |
| Nagaland | 736 |
| Orissa | 641 |
| Pondicherry | 302 |
| Punjab | 454 |
| Rajasthan | 1,153 |
| Sikkim | 8 |
| Tamil Nadu | 52,036 |
| Tripura | 5 |
| Uttar Pradesh | 1,751 |
| Uttranchal | 79 |
| West Bengal | 2,397 |
| Ahemdabad MC | 726 |
| Chennai MC | 0 |
| Mumbai MC | 10,362 |
| Total | 124,995 |

### HIV Statistics, 20051

The prevalence rates below are taken from data collected during screening of women attending antenatal clinics.

| State/Union Territory | HIV prevalence (%) |
|---|---|
| A & N Islands | 0.58 |
| Andhra Pardesh | 2.00 |
| Arunachal Pradesh | 0.43 |
| Assam | 0.00 |
| Bihar | 0.00 |
| Chandigarh | 0.00 |
| Chattisgarh | 0.25 |
| D & N Haveli | 0.30 |

*Contd...*

| State/Union Territory | HIV prevalence (%) |
|---|---|
| Daman & Diu | 0.13 |
| Delhi | 0.25 |
| Goa | 0.00 |
| Gujarat | 0.25 |
| Haryana | 0.13 |
| Himachal Pradesh | 0.13 |
| Jammu & Kashmir | 0.00 |
| Jharkhand | 0.13 |
| Karnataka | 1.25 |
| Kerala | 0.25 |
| Lakshdweep | 0.00 |
| Madhya Pardesh | 0.25 |
| Maharashtra | 1.25 |
| Manipur | 1.25 |
| Meghalaya | 0.00 |
| Mizoram | 0.88 |
| Nagaland | 1.63 |
| Orissa | 0.25 |
| Pondicherry | 0.25 |
| Punjab | 0.13 |
| Rajasthan | 0.13 |
| Sikkim | 0.30 |
| Tamil Nadu | 0.50 |
| Tripura | 0.00 |
| Uttar Pradesh | 0.00 |
| Uttranchal | 0.00 |
| West Bengal | 0.84 |

Some areas report an HIV prevalence rate of 0 in antenatal clinics. This does not necessarily mean that there is no HIV in the area, as some of them report the presence of the virus at

STD clinics and amongst injecting drug users. In many states and territories, the average antenatal HIV prevalence is based on reports from fewer than five clinics.

## AIDS FUELED BY ABUSES AGAINST CHILDREN

### *Children Affected by HIV/AIDS Face Lethal Discrimination and Exploitation*

India's explosive AIDS epidemic is being fueled by widespread abuses against children who are affected by HIV/AIDS, Human Rights Watch said in a new report released today. The Indian government's failure to address these abuses is undermining its anti-AIDS policy and putting millions of lives at risk.

Children are being turned away from schools, clinics and orphanages because they or their family members are HIV-positive. If the Indian government is serious about fighting the country's AIDS epidemic, it should stop ignoring children affected by AIDS and start protecting them from abuse. Zama Coursen-Neff, senior researcher with Human Rights Watch's Children's Rights Division

The 209-page report, "Future Forsaken: Abuses Against Children Affected by HIV/AIDS in India," documents that many doctors refuse to treat or even touch HIV-positive children. Some schools expel or segregate children because they or their parents are HIV-positive. Many orphanages and other residential institutions reject HIV-positive children or deny that they house them. Children from families affected by AIDS may be denied an education, pushed onto the street, forced into the worst forms of child labor, or otherwise exploited, all of which puts them at greater risk of contracting HIV.

"Children are being turned away from schools, clinics and orphanages because they or their family members are HIV-positive," said Zama Coursen-Neff, senior researcher with Human Rights Watch's Children's Rights Division and author of the report. "If the Indian government is serious about fighting the country's AIDS epidemic, it should stop ignoring children affected by AIDS and start protecting them from abuse."

In India hundreds of thousands of children are living with HIV/AIDS, according to official statistics. Children of parents with HIV/AIDS suffer in turn: many are forced to withdraw from school to care for sick parents, are forced to work to replace their parents' income, or are orphaned. Although the government has not conducted studies to assess the number of children affected by AIDS, some experts calculate that more than 1 million children under age 15 have lost one or both parents to HIV/AIDS. The Indian government estimates that 5.1 million people are living with HIV/AIDS in India.

Street children, child sex workers and children of sex workers, children from lower castes and Dalits (or "untouchables") suffer even more as they also face other forms of discrimination. Sexual abuse and violence against women and girls, coupled with their long-standing subordination in Indian society, make them especially vulnerable to HIV transmission. Girls are also more likely to be pulled out of school to care for a sick family member or to take over domestic work. When living with HIV/AIDS, they may be the last in the family to receive medical care.

Many children-and the professionals who care for them-are not getting the information about HIV they need to protect themselves or to combat discrimination. Fewer than half of all secondary schools offer any AIDS education. Those that do teach about HIV/AIDS do so at an age when most children, especially girls, have already dropped out. And the government is utterly failing to provide information to millions of India's children who are not in school but on the streets, at work, in institutions, in non-formal schools and at home.

"Children need accurate information to protect themselves from HIV/AIDS," said Coursen-Neff. "But the most vulnerable children are those who've dropped out of school, and they're the ones who are least likely to get lifesaving information about HIV prevention."

Misinformation and fear also cause some families to reject children who are HIV-positive or who are perceived to be. Although some state governments, like that of Tamil Nadu, have begun programs to educate the public, most have not.

"Many teachers, doctors, government officials and ordinary people in India still don't know the basic facts about HIV transmission and AIDS care," Coursen-Neff said.

In addition, many HIV-positive children are denied medical care because government facilities are either unavailable or lack basic medical supplies. Struggling families caring for HIV/AIDS-affected children find it even harder to pay school fees and related costs, further preventing some children from attending school.

Some government officials have started to speak out about the need to reach children who are seen to be "innocent victims." But children who face high risk of HIV, such as street children or child sex workers, are blamed for their "bad behavior" and their needs ignored. Human Rights Watch called on the Indian government to take immediate action to:

- Enact and enforce legislation proscribing discrimination against people living with HIV/AIDS. Among other things, such legislation should specify that children may never be barred from school solely because they are HIV-positive.
- Ensure that children living with HIV/AIDS receive all available medical care, including antiretroviral treatment.
- Address school fees and related costs that keep children, especially girls, from going to school. Children in school are generally less vulnerable to HIV/AIDS.
- Provide care and protection to children whose parents are unable to care for them because of HIV/AIDS.
- Provide all children, both in and out of school, with comprehensive, accurate and age-appropriate information about HIV/AIDS.

## FUTURE FORSAKEN: ABUSES AGAINST CHILDREN AFFECTED BY HIV/AIDS IN INDIA

"Anu P.," a 6-year-old in Maharashtra, was sent home from kindergarten in 2003 by her teacher, who instructed Anu's older sister to tell her "please not to come again to the school."

Her grandfather, who had been caring for Anu and her siblings after their parents died of AIDS, explained, "The teacher didn't allow her to come to school because she believes Anu is HIV-positive. I believe that other parents were talking amongst themselves, so the teacher said she shouldn't come." Her grandfather said he was afraid that if he protested, Anu's older sister might be sent away from school as well. A nearby private doctor told Anu's family not to bring the girl to his clinic "because if you do, other people won't come.'" The reason the man gave, her uncle said, was because of HIV. Anu's 66 year-old grandmother had been taking her on foot to the government hospital, but the distance had become too far for her to walk, her grandfather explained.

"Sharmila A.," age 10, was HIV-positive and had lost both of her parents to AIDS. She stopped going to school in the fourth grade. "When I went to school, I sat separately from the other children, in the last mat. I sat alone. The other children wanted to be with me, but the teacher would tell them not to play with me. She said, 'This disease will spread to you also, so do not play with her,'" Sharmila said. When she developed tuberculosis, she began traveling some four to five hours to reach a government-run hospital for free medical care. However, the hospital in Tamil Nadu did not provide antiretroviral drugs, and her health did not improve. Sharmila died in January 2004.

"Kannammal P." put her oldest daughter in an orphanage when she became unable to care for all of her children, she told us. Shortly thereafter, her husband was diagnosed with HIV. She went back to the orphanage and asked them for help. Instead, she said, "they asked the child to be tested, and then they wanted her to leave.... Despite pleading with the school authorities, they said, 'Sorry, please find another place. We are not free to take her.'" Her daughter's HIV test, she said, was negative. (AP) Sitting cross-legged on the cement floor of a home for abandoned children, 7-year-old Rupa-one of at least 60,000 Indian children infected with the AIDS virus-laughed excitedly, clicking the beads on an abacus.

"I've done it. I've won," she shouted, finishing her simple math problem ahead of a dozen other children crowding the sparsely furnished room. Rupa's bright eyes and high-spirited nature do not reflect her harrowing tale-of being shunned by neighbors and turned away from the homes of relatives when they learned she had tested positive for HIV, contracted at birth from her mother.

India and the United Nations have said 5.1 million adults are infected with the HIV virus here, the second-highest number in the world after South Africa.

Child sufferers are not included in that figure, but the government's AIDS control agency said 60,000 Indian children have the virus, while independent organizations have said the number may be closer to 100,000.

It was unclear how those numbers rank in comparison to other countries, but a report released Wednesday by Human Rights Watch said the Indian government is putting millions at risk by ignoring such children.

"Children affected by HIV/AIDS are being discriminated against in education and health services, denied care by orphanages, and pushed onto the streets and into the worst forms of child labor," Zama Coursen-Neff, the author of the report, told The Associated Press in an interview.

When a parent is infected, children drop out of school to care for them, or go to work to replace the lost income, until they become orphans, she said.

"Many doctors refuse to treat or even touch HIV-positive children," Human Rights Watch said. "Some schools expel or segregate children because they or their parents are HIV-positive."

## INDIAN CHILDREN IN THE NEW MILLENNIUM

The report urged the Indian government to adopt laws banning discrimination, specifically ensuring that no child is kept out of school. It also called on the state to care for all children whose parents are unable to provide for them because of the disease, and suggested an extensive public information campaign. In India, the virus initially infected prostitutes, their clients, drug addicts, and both homosexual and bisexual men. But it has spread to housewives, some of whom were infected by husbands who may have visited a prostitute or may be bisexual.

In a society where females are already undervalued-receiving less food, education and medical care-contracting the HIV virus is an additional burden because of the scarce resources available to them. This was evident in Rupa's case. Rupa's mother died of AIDS 10 years after she contracted the disease from her husband, who was a truck driver. Her two children were also infected.

"Rupa's younger brother, who has also tested positive, was taken back to the village by the children's father. But he left Rupa at our doorstep, saying the villagers would not welcome a girl child," said Doe Nair, head of the women's group that runs the children's home. Almost all the girls at the government-funded home have been abandoned by their families after testing positive for HIV, Nair said.

"The premium for a male child is so high in Indian society that families are ready to spend on his medical treatment and care," Nair said.

AIDS activists say young girls, orphaned after the death of their parents, are often thrown out of their homes and eventually pushed into prostitution.

At the mercy of pimps and brothel owners, they cannot insist that clients use a condom, said Anjali Gopalan, executive director of the Naz Foundation, a health agency that runs one of the few private clinics for AIDS patients in New Delhi.

"The discrimination that girls with HIV/AIDS face in the home, community and at the work place has remained largely invisible to government policy makers. There are no programs that focus on their problems," said Kousalya Perisamy of the Positive Women Network, an activist group working in southern Tamil Nadu state.

Meenakshi Dutta-Ghosh, who heads the Indian government's National AIDS Control Organization, said the government may have ignored children with HIV in the past, but she argued that health authorities have refocused their prevention and care programs in the last two years. "Earlier, for whatever reason, children were not a priority. This has changed. We are looking at children and young people as a category of focused attention," Dutta-Ghosh said.

The government had not given a figure for the number of child victims before, but Dutta-Ghosh offered the 60,000 estimate in an interview this week.

She said the government was working with independent groups and state welfare programs to reach children outside the regular school network, including street children, dropouts and child prostitutes.

But Gopalan called for laws to require protection of children with the disease. "There has to be a sustained effort at sensitizing officials, doctors, teachers, people at all levels," she said. "There's a long battle ahead."

## LETHAL DISCRIMINATION AND EXPLOITATION

India's explosive AIDS epidemic is being fuelled bywidespread abuses against children who are affected by HIV/AIDS, Human Rights Watchsaid in a new report released today. The Indian government's failure to address these abuses is undermining its anti-AIDS policy and putting millions of lives at risk. The 209-page report, "Future Forsaken: Abuses Against Children Affected by HIV/AIDS in India," documents that many doctors refuse to treat or even touch HIV-positive children. Some schools expel or segregate children because they or their parents are HIV-positive. Many orphanages and other residential institutions reject HIV-positive children or deny that they house them.

Children from families affected by AIDS maybe denied an education, pushed onto the street, forced into the worst forms of child labour, or otherwise exploited, all of which puts them at greater risk of contracting HIV. In India hundreds of thousands of children are living with HIV/AIDS, according to official statistics. Children of parents with HIV/AIDS suffer in turn: many are forced to withdraw from school to care for sick parents, are forced to work to replace their parents' income, or are orphaned. Although the government has not conducted studies to assess the number of children affected by AIDS, some experts calculate that more than 1 million children under age 15 have lost one or both parents to HIV/AIDS. The Indian government estimates that 5.1 million people are living with HIV/AIDS in India. Street children, child sex workers and children of sex workers, children from lower castes and Dalits (or "untouchables") suffer even more as they also face other forms of discrimination.

Sexual abuse and violence against women and girls, coupled with their long-standing subordination in Indian society, make them especially vulnerable to HIV transmission. Girls are also more likely to be pulled out of school to care for a sick family member or to take over domestic work. When living with HIV/AIDS, they may be the last in the family to receive medical care. Many children-and the professionals who care for them-are not getting the information about HIV they need to protect themselves or to combat discrimination. Fewer than half of all secondary schools offer any AIDS education. Those that do teach about HIV/AIDS do so at an age when most children, especially girls, have already dropped out. And the government is utterly failing to provide information to millions of India's children who are not in school but on the streets, at work, in institutions, in non-formal schools and at home.

## HELPING INDIAN CHILDREN WITH AIDS

### Partnership for a Better Life

Two little girls had lost their parents. Then they learned they have AIDS. No one wants them.

An alarming 90 percent of the 5.1 million people in India infected with HIV/AIDS don't know they have contracted the HIV virus that causes AIDS until a crisis occurs. So when a parent dies unexpectedly or a newborn becomes ill, HIV/AIDS is often discovered to be the cause. After that, the community frequently becomes frightened and shuns the family. Relatives will not take the children in. Schools reject them.

"The stigma is the challenge," said Dr. Pinagapany Manorama, of Chennai (formerly known as Madras), India. Inspired by the two girls who had AIDS but nowhere to turn,

Dr. Manorama created Chennai's Community Health Education Society (CHES), an organization that finds resources to house, educate and nurture shunned children. Supported by the U.S. Agency for International Development (USAID), CHES operates five family resource centers where people learn how to care for stricken families and where myths and misinformation about HIV/AIDS are corrected to reduce fear and slow the spread of the disease. A separate CHES shelter houses and educates 32 AIDS-affected children who have nowhere to live and no family to turn to.

Thanks to interventions by CHES, one young resident of the CHES orphanage, Murugan, won a watch for being the top student at his school—one of the few that accepts children affected by HIV/AIDS. At a CHES community resource center, two adolescent peer counselors plan for a street performance about HIV/AIDS while a community educator meets with a self-help group. Many of the CHES staff are HIV-positive.

Dr. Manorama's desire to help the two girls continues to have a ripple effect in the community, each day helping more and more people affected by HIV/AIDS live with dignity and respect.

### HIV Positive Children to get Access to Treatment

**New Delhi, 30th November 2006:** The Government of India, through the National AIDS Control Organization, in collaboration with the Indian Academy of Pediatricians, UNICEF, WHO and the Clinton Foundation HIV/AIDS Initiative today launched a National Pediatric Programme on HIV/AIDS. The first phase of the programme aims to put 10 000 children on ART treatment for life.

This initiative was inaugurated by Smt. Sonia Gandhi at the newly opened Anti Retroviral Therapy Center for children at the Kalavati Saran Children's Hospital in New Delhi today.

In her address, Smt. Sonia Gandhi said that we had come a long way since the Unite for Children and Unite Against Aids campaign which was inaugurated by President Kalam on 25th October 2005 as today a number of children will have access to life saving ART. Smt. Sonia Gandhi expressed concern about the discrimination faced by HIV+ people, especially women and children in rural areas and urged everyone present in the auditorium and NGOs and CBOs to fight against it. Smt. Sonia Gandhi congratulated the National AIDS Control Organization, Indian Academy of Pediatricians, UNICEF, WHO and the Clinton Foundation for doing an excellent job on National Pediatric Programme on HIV/AIDS.

Speaking on the rationale of the programme, Mr. William J. Clinton said that worldwide nearly 11,000 people are infected daily by HIV and children are a significant number. Large numbers of HIV infected children have no access to treatment due to lack of awareness and availability of drugs. The partnership in India is a significant achievement and a positive step to address access to treatment. The main purpose of the programme is to assist the government in treatment of children infected with HIV/AIDS.

In India it is estimated that 202,000 children are infected by HIV/AIDS (UNAIDS 2004). Using a conservative transmission rate of 30% from an infected mother to child, a new group of children of approximately 56,700 HIV infected are born every year (NACO, 2005). Global experience shows that 25-30% of children, who acquire HIV from their mothers die before their first birthday. Most of them (50-60%) will develop symptoms early in life and, in absence of timely diagnosis and anti-retroviral therapy and general HIV care, the progression of HIV infection in children is particularly aggressive.

In order to prolong happy and healthy life for children living with HIV, the Government of India, through the National AIDS Control Organization launched this National Pediatric Programme on HIV/AIDS. As a result, all children who were exposed to HIV will be tested for infection, a CD 4 cell estimation test will be performed to assess the stage of the decease progression and treatment will be advised if they are found to be requiring the treatment. Since September 2006 children across five states (Tamil Nadu, Andra Pradesh, Mahrashtra, Karnataka, and Delhi) have been mobilized, screened and if appropriate put on treatment. To date, the number of children who are on ART since the drive initiated is 3600. This access will be broadened to encompass the entire country.

National AIDS Control Programme (NACO) Director General, Ms. K Sujatha Rao, said, "This initiative is significant in addressing the need for treatment in children. Under the NACP III the aim is that there would be a universal access to treatment by the year 2011. The primary target is to place 10,000 children on treatment by March 2007."

Today, the National Pediatric Anti Retroviral Therapy (ART) Treatment and Dosing Guidelines developed by IAP with support from WHO, UNICEF and Clinton Foundation were also released. UNICEF has provided technical support to ensure quality roll out of the programme and will continue to monitor both coverage and quality.

The first phase of this initiative includes training of pediatricians and counselors, establishing laboratory diagnosis, introducing Dried Blood Spot system to transport dried blood samples and procure paediatric Anti retroviral drugs and Cotrimaxazole. The impact of treatment can be seen within six moths of initiation. There is a dramatic positive change in the before and after scenario. The child is thriving, cheerful, puts on weight and returns to normal childhood. As a result, there already has been a good response to the drive and a positive network representative said that "The children are responding well to ART. Earlier they used to have many medical problems like fever, diarrhea etc. Now they are healthy and we are very happy with the fact that now children are getting treatment." Clinton Foundation will supplement the treatment with care and support services to children.

The initiative has set up a unique partnership between the technical agencies and the NGO's and networks of positive people under the stewardship of NACO.

### School Teachers Awarded for Imparting Knowledge on HIV/AIDS amongst Students

**New Delhi, December 01, 2006:** In a unique initiative to felicitate school teachers towards their efforts for implementing Adolescence Education Programme (AEP) and imparting knowledge on HIV/AIDS amongst young school students, the Hon'ble Minister of State for Education awarded 25 teachers from 10 states of India-New Delhi, Orissa, Madhya Pradesh,

Bihar, Chattisgarh, Maharashtra, Tamil Nadu, Karnataka, Andhra Pradesh and Rajasthan, acknowledging their contribution.

Applauding teachers for their efforts, M.A.A Fatmi, Hon'ble Minister of state for Education and Literacy, said "It gives me immense pleasure to recognize teachers who are making this significant contribution to the cause of HIV/AIDS. India has growing young population as well as growing number of HIV/AIDS cases. Therefore, it is important to educate the young school students on issues pertaining to HIV/AIDS and provide them with correct information on the same. And who would be better than Teacher/Guru to impart this knowledge."

The Adolescence Education Programme is positioned by the Department of Education and the National AIDS Control Organisation (NACO) in partnership with UNESCO, UNICEF & UNFPA, as a key intervention in preventing new HIV infections and reducing social vulnerability to the infection. The programme is implemented in all states across the country through the Department of Education (DoE) in collaboration with the State AIDS Control Societies (SACS).

Excited on the success of the Adolescence Education Programme, Mr. Eimar Barr, Deputy Director (Programmes), UNICEF, India, said, "The basic idea behind implementing the programme was to help fight the HIV epidemic and change people's attitude towards those living with HIV. The objective was to provide adequate and accurate knowledge about HIV in the context of life-skills. The programme aimed at educating young people about themselves, their sexuality and adolescence. The program also encapsulates facts on HIV and other sexually transmitted infections, enabling them to protect themselves, dispel myths and clarify misconceptions. Emphasis was also laid on life skill approach program, where the session focused on ways to contribute to the well being of the young and empower them meet many challenges of life. "

The programme was conducted by teachers of Government schools across the country, who were trained to understand the issues pertaining to the subject and address them accordingly. According to the study conducted, there was an increase of 86%

in coverage target in 2005-06, equipping more than 10 million adolescents with information and skills in HIV prevention. To facilitate the Teachers Awards/Recognition system, UNICEF contracted ORG Marg to assess teachers from 8000 schools across 10 states. The assessment survey consisted of anonymous questionnaire that was circulated amongst students. The key parameters on which teachers were assessed: innovativeness in their practices in classroom, confidentiality with students on their queries, thorough knowledge on the subject and the most approachable teacher.

Providing details of the Teachers Awards/Recognition system, Ms. K. Sujatha Rao, Director General, National Aids Control Organization, said, "The incidence of HIV/AIDS is increasing among young people. We recognize that working with and helping them understand issues pertaining to HIV/ AIDS, is critical to arrest this disease."

"Based on the preliminary analysis conducted in 2005, it was found that teachers are the most effective communicators of information regarding HIV prevention, as students are still reticent in speaking on Sexuality and Growing up Issues. Keeping these findings in view, we decided to liaise with teachers across school in India to facilitate the same."

The Adolescence Education programme is positioned by the Department of Education and the National AIDS Control Organisation as a key intervention in preventing new HIV infections and reducing social vulnerability to the infection. The programme was implemented in all states across the country through the Department of Education in collaboration with the State AIDS Control Societies.

The Adolescence Education programme is being conducted by teachers, where they educated students about different aspects of HIV, i.e., growing up & Adolescence, Sexually transmitted Infection & HIV/AIDS and skills for HIV protection.

Emphasis was also laid on Life Skill Programme. The life skill approach/Programme addresses young people ages 14 onwards and aims to strengthen their knowledge and life skills to enable them to effectively cope with risky situation they encounter in their daily lives. The life skills program was designed to enable youngsters to make positive health choices, make informed choices, develop supportive relationship with trusted care-givers (parents, community members), practice healthy behaviours and recognize and avoid risky health situations

The Adolescence Education programme also aims to support Young People's Right to know about themselves, their adolescence and their sexuality, basic facts on HIV and other sexually transmitted infections, develop and reinforce life skills that enables them to protect themselves, dispel myths and clarify misconceptions and find ways where they can help fight the HIV epidemic and encourage positive attitudes towards people living with HIV.

## HIV/AIDS IN INDIA

The first case of HIV/AIDS was reported in Tamil Nadu, India in 1986. Since then the virus has spread from the high risk groups to the general population very fast. Today, there are 5.7 million people living with HIV/AIDS in India.

### Women and Children

Women and children are increasingly becoming vulnerable to HIV/AIDS. The new findings conclude that 38% of the infected persons in India are women. The male-female ratio of infected people shifted from 55 per 100 males in 2001 to 60 in 2005. This indicates the increasing feminization of HIV/AIDS in India.

This alarming trend is being observed closely as more HIV positive mothers will unknowingly pass the virus on to their children. The incidence of parent to child transmission jumped from 2.7% to 3.5% in just one year. India has an estimated 2.2 million children infected by HIV/AIDS. As of July 2006, about 1,850 children were receiving ART in India. NACO with support of Indian Academy of Pediatrics, Clinton Foundation, UNICEF and WHO have formulated the policy and guidelines which form the basis of the "National Paediatric initiative" for children living with HIV. NACO under this initiative has set a target for providing Anti Retroviral Therapy (ART) to 10,000 children in 2006-07. This initiative has been launched on 30th November by Mrs. Sonia Gandhi and William. J. Clinton.

## Young People

Over 35% of AIDS cases reported are below 25 years of age and 50% of new infections are between 15 and 24 years old. The current HIV/AIDS programmes are reaching only 15% of young people and 17% of high risk group sub-population such as sex workers, men who have sex with men and injecting drug users. Less than one quarter of young people have accurate information on how to protect themselves from HIV which, coupled with profound gender inequalities, make change in sexual attitudes and practices very difficult. It is estimated that there are 200 million young people in high prevalence and highly vulnerable districts who need access to information, skills and services to reduce their vulnerability to HIV infection.

Primary prevention among young people is the greatest hope to change the course of the epidemic in India. As a result, the Adolescent Education Programme has been conceived by UNICEF, NACO, Ministry of Education, UNESCO and UNFPA. The programme is implemented in all states across the country through the Department of Education (DoE) in collaboration with the State AIDS Control Societies (SACS).

This programme aims at 100% coverage of schools by 2006-7 (33 million students every academic year). The curriculum includes growing up, HIV/AIDS, life skills and extra curricular activities. Already, 110,000 of the 150,000 high schools in India trained teachers and peer educators to pass on life skills and preventive messages.

On 1st December 25 best performing teachers were given national awards for imparting knowledge of HIV/AIDS amongst students.

## Communications and Advocacy

Communications and advocacy on HIV/AIDS is essential to break the silence and contain the spread of the decease. To achieve this, UNICEF works on two levels: (1) Promote HIV/AIDS awareness among young people and empower them to take collective action to fight against HIV/AIDS. (2) Influence the policy-makers and key stakeholders at national, state and district levels to influence the policy, promote multi-sectoral response and increase government resources to fight against HIV/AIDS.

**Unite for Children Unite Against AIDS:** UNICEF has been carrying out focused popular campaigns to raise awareness among the children and young people through Unite for children Unite Against AIDS.

This campaign calls upon everyone to join together to put the care and protection of children, adolescents and young people at the centre of the HIV/AIDS agenda. Specifically, the campaign will work to mobilize resources, foster corporate social responsibility, move toward universal access to antiretroviral treatment, reduce the price of existing treatment and testing.

UNICEF popular campaigns are supported by famous celebrities from all walks of life, including films, sports, faith networks, political leaders and positive networks themselves.

This year, during the Championship Trophy, world cricket teams have taken up the issues of HIV/AIDS and delivered Public Service Announcements (PSAs). Through these PSAs world famous cricketers asked children and young people to learn more about HIV/AIDS and protect themselves and people around them form HIV infection and respect people who are HIV+. The South African team went a bit further and got involved in a special programme with HIV+ children in Gujarat.

**Policy and Advocacy:** UNICEF works hand in hand with the Government of India through NACO in order to influence the HIV/AIDS policies. Currently UNICEF is influencing the new HIV/AIDS Bill to make sure that children and women are well represented and HIV infected and affected children are granted with all rights on par with grown up adults.

## HIV/AIDS

With an estimated 4.58 million HIV positive cases, India has the second largest number of people in the world living with HIV. This accounts for 11.4 per cent of global HIV infections.

The epidemic is unevenly distributed across India, with just six states accounting for 80 per cent of the estimated cases: Andhra Pradesh, Karnataka, Maharashtra, Manipur, Nagaland

and Tamil Nadu. In these states, the HIV prevalence rate among women attending antenatal clinics exceeds 1 per cent-an indication that the epidemic has spread from high-risk groups, such as sex workers and injecting drug users, to the general population.

The main mode of HIV transmission is through sexual contact. The exception is in the north-eastern states of Manipur and Nagaland, where injecting drug use accounts for the majority of the transmission.

Awareness and knowledge of prevention are crucial to checking the spread of HIV. In 2001 a behaviour surveillance survey (BSS) conducted by the National AIDS Control Organisation (NACO) indicated increased levels of awareness but also revealed that very few people correctly understood how to prevent transmission.

Fewer than half of all people interviewed were aware of the two important methods of prevention of transmission: consistent condom use and sexual relationships with faithful and uninfected partners. Awareness is especially low amongst women. The survey found that while 70 per cent of men were aware of the protective value of a condom, only 48 per cent of women knew about this. The epidemic is shifting towards women and young people, with women accounting for 25 per cent of all HIV infections. Low levels of awareness, spiralling violence within the home and limited access to health-care are also responsible for the growing incidence of HIV/AIDS amongst women. Stigma and discrimination continue to be among the biggest barriers to prevention, care and treatment.

## GLOBAL AIDS-INDIA

### Indian Children with HIV-July 7, 2003

The impact of the HIV epidemic on children has been complex and diverse. The stigma and discrimination faced by persons living with HIV/AIDS (PLHAs) is compounded in the case of children. Children and youth are physiologically more vulnerable to contracting HIV than adults, particularly when they are subject to sexual abuse, and a child's chances of losing both parents relatively quickly are far higher where the parents are PLHAs. Recognising that the effect of HIV/AIDS is not limited to children who have lost their parents to the epidemic, 'children affected by HIV/AIDS' are recognised as those having a parent or guardian living with HIV/AIDS, those having lost a parent or guardian to AIDS, those living in households fostering children orphaned by AIDS, or those who are themselves living with HIV/AIDS.

Further the notion of 'AIDS orphans' has been expanded to include children below the age of 18 who have lost one or both their parents to AIDS.

Laws relating to children in India remain paternalistic, based on the view that persons below a certain age do not possess the ability to make certain decisions. This view is reinforced by providing an age bar for marriage, contracts etc. In most Indian laws persons below the age of 18 are referred to as minors. However, this does not account for age-specific needs of children and adolescents in the context of HIV/AIDS.

The law must recognise that the participation of young persons, especially adolescents, in decisions and interventions that affect them, is integral to the success of any HIV/AIDS intervention and to provide sensitive and appropriate support and treatment to young persons affected by HIV/AIDS.

**Consent for Testing and Confidentiality**

Issues of primary concern for children affected by HIV/AIDS relate to mandatory testing policies and the preservation of confidentiality.

For children and adolescents, this is problematic as they are not recognised as persons who can or should have access to sexual or general health services without a guardian. Not only does this restrict the rights of children in general, the system also does not account for a large percentage of children who live and work outside family structures.

Legal strategies in other countries have been reformed accordingly to empower children (by specifying requirements in terms of age and the ability of the child to understand the nature of the diagnosis or treatment) to consent to testing and provide them the same rights as adults vis-à-vis confidentiality.

The issue of confidentiality for minors also arises in educational/institutional settings. Generally, information regarding the HIV status of a minor or her/his parents cannot be shared and should be disclosed based only on pre-determined protocols.

Children in institutional care are frequently subjected to mandatory testing, breach of their HIV status and discrimination. Legislation should outline the circumstances in which minors in institutional care who are incapable of understanding the nature of the diagnosis or treatment can be tested and also protect their right to confidentiality.

## Discrimination

The impact of HIV/AIDS related discrimination is significantly felt by children in educational and institutional settings such as orphanages, juvenile homes etc. This issue has been highlighted by the recent expulsion of two HIV positive children from a school in Kerala.

Traditional discriminatory practices in India such as the refusal to treat adolescents, the denial of sexual health information, the promotion of abstinence only approaches, perpetuation of gender and sexual stereotypes have put minors, especially youth, at an increased risk to HIV.

International law, judgements and research have recognised the need for adolescents to access sexual health information and have affirmed their right to receive age appropriate sexual and health information, including condoms.

## Children in Different Settings

Indian law does not, as such, deal with child specific issues in civil or criminal laws and children's issues have been discussed mostly in the context of child labour and child marriages. Unlike other jurisdictions Indian law does not recognise the child as separate from her/his guardians or parents. This limited understanding prevents children from accessing sexual health information and services. The Indian legal paradigm should enable children and adolescents to exercise their rights in different situations.

The paper highlights some of the issues particular to the settings in which children find themselves. Thus children in families may face issues relating to inheritance, property rights, guardianship and adoption. Children living with or affected by HIV/AIDS in India are commonly discriminated against in schools and in many cases, schools refuse to accept children as students because they are HIV-positive or their parents are HIV positive.

Similarly, children living and working on the streets or within informal structures face discrimination at different levels that not only affect their ability to protect themselves from HIV, but in fact increase their vulnerability significantly.

One of the key factors responsible for transmission of the HIV virus to a child is child sexual abuse. In India, 47% to 76% of children, especially girls, have reported sexual abuse. However, the law in India still provides no deterrent to child sexual abusers in the form of punishment and does not in fact specifically recognise the crime of child sexual abuse.

## State Protection, Institutionalisation and Minors

The Indian State has interpreted its protective role for children and minors living outside family structures or in violent situations as limited to providing for their institutionalisation.

This policy has contributed significantly to discrimination as it places minors in extreme positions of powerlessness. For instance, where children come in conflict with the law, the provisions of the Juvenile Justice Act 2000 are applicable. Under this law, the juvenile justice system has the power to test a child for HIV without her/his consent. Further there are no safeguards to protect medical records and the child can be isolated on the basis of her/his HIV-positive status. Such policies fail to recognise that encouraging (and recognising) the collectivisation of children/youth, providing relevant education and skills, creating accessible sexual health information and health services etc. may in fact be more effective in empowering children/youth than displacing them from their environment.

It is only after this re-conceptualisation that effective strategies can be put in place to change the circumstances which make children and young people vulnerable to exploitation, violence and HIV.

The rights of children have been the subject matter of several international conventions and guidelines. The Convention on the Rights of the Child is the most widely acceded international convention which recognises the rights of the child and the obligations of the State towards children.

These obligations have expanded in the HIV/AIDS context. This paper argues that the recognition of these rights demands both legislative and policy initiatives for children living with HIV/AIDS and AIDS orphans.

Such initiatives include community based integrationist programs, incorporation of standards of care in institutions, providing access to the legal system, and changes in laws, particularly criminal laws (to address child sexual abuse and violence).

Children With HIV/AIDS Neglected in India. ( News Report From The Hindu).

According to UNAIDS, 120,000 Indian children were living with the HIV virus in 2004. The National AIDS Control Organisation (NACO) estimated that around 60,000 new infections occurred last year and activists estimate that around 250,000 Indian children are HIV-positive today but there is no accurate estimate. On May 31, 2006, at the United Nations General Assembly Special Session (UNGASS) in New York to review the 2001 Declaration on HIV/AIDS-the Indian delegation's report included commitments to prepare by 2003 and implement by 2005 strategies for special assistance for children orphaned by, and vulnerable to, HIV/AIDS, reduce the number of infections passed from mother to child by 20 per cent, and roll out treatment and care. Examining the progress made reveals that though the present government has recognised the need to give adequate attention to HIV/AIDS, children in India remain the forgotten face. No national strategy currently exists to aid children affected by HIV.

The national AIDS Control Organization (NACO) concedes that it has made no progress in designing and implementing programmes for children vulnerable to HIV but Dr. Sujatha Rao, director-general of NACO, has said that these children will be accorded greater priority in the next National AIDS Control Programme, NACP III. This will include livelihood support and education provisions. However, it is not clear whether they will be provided with proper treatment. No India-specific guidelines for the treatment, care, and support of children living with HIV have been distributed so far. Government centres administer paediatric dosages of antiretroviral (ARV) drugs based on World Health Organisation recommendations by weight band.

This is problematic because children's bodies absorb and metabolise drugs differently. Although India-specific guidelines have been prepared by the Indian Academy of Paediatricians, sources say these have not yet reached the NACO national network. As of April, only 1,215 of the NACO-estimated 39,000 children who need ARVs were receiving them, a document prepared by the International Treatment Preparedness Coalition (ITPC) stated. According to K.K. Abraham, president of the Indian Network for People Living with HIV/AIDS (INP+), these dosages may still be administered by dividing fractions of adult formulations, which often leads to under or over dosage through human error, and over time, drug resistance. Since the national programme does not yet administer second line drugs free of charge, it would seem that any child who develops immunity has a short future. There are no paediatric medical formulations available under the government-sponsored programme.

Until last year, some of the best tools used in the fight against HIV in adults were not available for children at affordable prices. "Now, there are at least 15 paediatric drugs that have been approved for use by WHO, and six of those drugs are made in India," said Vineeta Gupta, director of Stop HIV/AIDS in India Initiative (SHAII), a Washington-based NRI advocacy group. Two paediatric three-in-one dose combinations available: are Emtri (zidovudine/lamivudine/nevirapine), manufactured by Emcure, and Triomune (stavudine/lamivudine/nevirapine), manufactured by Cipla. Both have Indian Regulatory Drug approval. Emtri is already in use in Africa, Latin America, and Asia.

Triomune is being marketed to private hospitals and NGOs. Although NACO has licensed State AIDS Control Societies in Tamil Nadu, West Bengal, Mumbai, and Varanasi to procure paediatric drugs independently, none is provided under the national programme.

India's National AIDS Control Organization, which this month is scheduled to launch the third phase of its National AIDS Control Program, plans to provide 300,000 HIV-positive adults and 40,000 children ages 15 and younger living with the virus with access to no-cost antiretroviral drugs, the Indian Express reports. NACO during its second phase provided treatment access to 65,000 HIV-positive adults, and the organization since December 2006 has provided 3,700 HIV-positive children with treatment access, the Express reports. According to the Express, NACO has increased the number of health centers that provide no-cost antiretrovirals from 56 to 120 (Batra Bakshi, Indian Express, 3/31). Under NACO's third phase, the Indian government also aims to collaborate with private sector health care providers to offer HIV/AIDS treatment to an additional seven million people, including high-risk and impoverished populations. NACP estimates that because at least 75,000 to one million HIV-positive people will seek care in the private sector, an additional 126 antiretroviral drug treatment centers will be needed nationwide (Kaiser Daily HIV/AIDS Report, 1/4).

According to Confederation of Indian Industry Chief Mentor Tarun Das, CII members plan to spend $23 million to establish 100 additional health facilities that offer access to no-cost antiretrovirals during NACO's third phase. Das added that over 1,000 companies affiliated with the Associated Chambers of Commerce and Industry of India have agreed to follow the guidelines for the control of HIV/AIDS at workplaces.

## STOP HIV/AIDS IN INDIA

Association for Indias Development (MD), in partnership with Insaaf International and International Commission of Jurists (Punjab), is initiating a coordinated global effort to organize people and organizations concerned with social justice and health for all to Stop HIV/AIDS in India. This effort is focused on HIV/AIDS, Malaria and Tuberculosis. The first step is to stop the Amendment to the Patents Act of 1970, soon to come before Indian Parliament. To stop implementation of the Ordinance to amend the Patents Act followed by Amendment to the Patents Act is more urgent and needed in light of Tsunami Disaster. The price hike of the medicines will have short term and long term adverse effects for the relief work and rehabilitation efforts in the region.

We call upon all people and organizations to join us in this endeavor by: Signing and disseminating a petition to be submitted to the Government of India through the Indian Embassy in Washington D.C. The petition is available at:

What this amended Patents Act would do: It would adversely affect the availability, accessibility and affordability of medicines thus undermining the right to health. The impacts of the proposed amendment amount to the violation of national and international human rights obligations including the International Covenant on Economic Social and Cultural Rights, Indias Protection of Human Rights Act (1993), Alma Ata Declaration (1978), and the People's Charter for Health (2000). If adopted, India would be trading away its own right to protect public health, as well as the rights of people in other poor countries.

India would no longer be able to produce affordable generic medicines. This especially would affect HIV medicines for second line treatment. The cost of annual treatment in these cases would jump from $250 a year to $700-$3000.

The prices of medicines would shoot up and would affect the millions of people suffering from a wide range of life-threatening and chronic diseases, which including not only HIV infection but also tuberculosis, diabetes, respiratory tract infections, and various forms of cancer.

It would have global repercussions as India plays a unique role in global access to medicines. India is the world's chief exporter of affordable generic drugs, especially to Africa and Asia. This amendment would threaten the survival of millions of indigent people with HIV in these regions. The proposed Bill would introduce product patents in the fields of food, chemicals, and pharmaceuticals. The product patents would cost both the economy and the consumer heavily. The domestic small-scale industry, a once-promised feature of the dream of a self-reliant, independent India, would further lose ground to unequal competition from multi-national companies.

It is your cause:

**If You are Concerned about Increasing HIV/AIDS:** The gigantic challenge to stop HIV/AIDS in the world requires a concerted effort from all of us. Worldwide, 60-70 million people have been infected with HIV. Each year 3 million people die of AIDS, including 500,000 children and the disease is an expanding pandemic. Many experts believe India is the decisive battleground in the fight against the disease.

**If You are Concerned about Equality and Health Rights:** Poor people are more prone to communicable diseases and stand to lose the most with rising drug prices. Healthcare will increasingly become a privilege of the rich. Health rights for all irrespective of socio-economic status is promised by the Indian constitution and international human rights norms and yet it is not provided. The struggle for actualization would suffer a serious and grave setback.

**If You are Concerned about Gender Equality and Women's Empowerment:** Gender discrimination and lack of female empowerment is a significant risk factor for contracting HIV/AIDS. Women have little power to negotiate safer sexual practices and have little access to family resources. Thus, they will suffer most from rising costs of the medicines.

**If You are Concerned about International Financial Institutions Putting Profits over People:** For several years, India resisted pressure from the WTO to amend its Patents Act of 1970. Under an ultimatum from the WTO, India promulgated an ordinance to bring about the changes in its Patents Act. If not stopped, the same changes will become law within the next six months.

**If You are Concerned about India, its People, and Poor People Across the Globe:** Indias present Patents Law allows production of affordable and generic medicines. Not only in India, but elsewhere in other developing countries, poor people benefit from these medicines. UNICEF has stated that there are signs of a rapidly-spreading AIDS epidemic in India. Home to the world's second-largest HIV-positive population with an estimated 5.1 million people living with HIV/AIDS, India acquires nearly 1000 new cases per month. Poor people need generics.

**If You are Concerned about People Dying from Preventable Causes and Diseases:** Anti-retroviral drugs are required to prevent HIV especially in mother-to-child transmission. They will become unaffordable not only in India but also in other developing nations. Most of the medicines will be at least 99% more expensive than they are now. That means more disease, suffering, and mortality. India is already facing the challenge of an increase in resistant tuberculosis and mutant strains of malarial parasite. Affordable medicine can deal with this threat.

## A CHILD-FRIENDLY KIT FOR HIV/AIDS AWARENESS

The special kit named HAAP will help in creating awareness on HIV/AIDS in India and countering the social stigma attached with the disease. Developed in four languages namely Hindi, English, Telugu and Kannada, HAAP will enable children to learn about HIV/AIDS. It disseminates information through puppets, comic books, computer games and animation films. Scores of children participated in the launch of the innovative child-friendly communication tool kit on HIV/AIDS awareness this Wednesday in the capital. A core team comprising of representatives of Plan India, DFID, UNAIDS visited five different states of Delhi, Rajasthan, Karnataka, Maharashtra and Andhra Pradesh and conducted residential workshops with the children. "It is a child-friendly communication tool in order to disseminate messages on HIV/AIDS awareness in order to reduce stigma and discrimination," said Bhagyashree Dengle, Executive Director, Plan India. Teenagers and youngsters in the age group of twelve to sixteen hailing from diverse backgrounds participated in the creation and development of "HAAP". Individual experts motivated these children to attempt such a novel task and provided the technical know-how about the content and story-lines. "I learnt a lot about HIV/AIDS from this initiative. I learnt how it spreads and what steps should be taken to prevent it.

I was also sensitized on how to behave with patients suffering from HIV/AIDS," said Ashish Kumar, a student. At present about 1,000 HAAP kits have been prepared and another 5,000 kits are in the pipeline. The kits will be distributed across India in schools and self-help groups to reach out to greater audience and help in bringing a change the general outlook towards HIV/AIDS patients. "That is a great initiative. It is fantastic to see the development of tools of communication, which are adapted to children, which are developed by children themselves so that they can explain to other children how to resist the stigma against HIV.

I think it is a very important development," said Denis Broun, Country Head, UNAIDS. The approach behind the whole programme is to promote children as agents of change in society rather than mere recipients. Plan India has taken up the cause of pediatric AIDS in India after cases of discrimination against children suffering from HIV/AIDS started cropping up. According to UNAIDS, 60,000 infants suffering with AIDS are born every year in the country. According to the United Nations, 5.7 million Indians are living with HIV/AIDS-the world's largest case-load.

## Five Questions on HIV/AIDS in India

I was recently asked the following five questions following India's first National Parliamentarians Forum on HIV/AIDS held on 25-26 July 2003 in New Delhi. At this meeting roughly one thousand members from the state and central governments met to plan a cohesive and effective response to the spread of this deadly scourge. The convention was addressed by the Prime Minister, many other prominent ministers, and Dr. Peter Piot, head of UNAIDS. Here are my thoughts on the questions asked.

1. Do you think that India is deprived of international attention for its HIV/AIDS problem because countries like South Africa get more news headlines? If so, do you think this has contributed to the spread of disease?

While sex workers, truckers, MSM have been the buzz words, four factors have been the major contributors to the spread of HIV/AIDS in India. They are (i) the lack of a health care and education system that reaches and serves all people; (ii) marginalized and poor populations, (iii) risky sexual behaviors, and (iv) IV drug use. To ameliorate these four problems, international organizations and outside nations can draw attention to the problem, suggest intervention strategies, and provide seed resources to help implement them. The local governments (central and states) have to create the infrastructure, enact enabling laws, and commit resources; the bureaucracy has to assume responsibility for implementation; the medical community has to turn it into another chronic, expensive, terminal but manageable disease; the education system has to teach a curriculum on reproductive health, sexuality, sex, sexually transmitted diseases, and drug addiction before children start experimenting with these; condoms have be available freely, widely and easily; and the society has to overcome its irrational fears and remove stigma, discrimination and exploitation.

I believe India has enough intelligent people to understand the devastation in Sub-Saharan Africa, the reasons for international attention and funding, and the impact of the growing numbers. So I believe that international attention has made the intelligentsia aware. The reason they have not responded is not because they have not been told, but because strategic thinking is missing, narrow self-interests dominate thinking and action, and those in power and with money believe they will escape the devastation. Health is not a focus of the government, health ministries languish in political backwaters, health ministers without any background in health come and go, and these failings continue. I doubt if international agencies can "fix" these problems of India.

As regards international funding, almost all funding for HIV/AIDS intervention in India is from outside. I believe that unless India commits its own resources and takes ownership for solving the problem, they will not be able to stem the tide. Money, by any means, has become central to most [urban] Indians, especially to the politicians, therefore only by committing their own resources will India demonstrate it is ready to act. For those who claim there is no money, one must not forget that the government was able to INCREASE the defence budget by almost INR 120 billion (nine times the central government's budget on health) after the Kargil fiasco in 1999! So, clearly, health continues to NOT be a national priority.

Given the magnitude of the world-wide spread, how different countries are at different stages of the pandemic and have different levels of ability and resources to respond, it is difficult to expect international agencies to solve India's problem. India is of great historical, cultural, geographical, economic and strategic value to the world but the reality is it has to solve its own problems, especially that of HIV/AIDS. So I would put 90% of the responsibility on the shoulders of the Indian elite for choosing not to respond and 10% on international agencies for not being more involved.

2. Do you think education about AIDS is getting through to the general population? What barriers are there to effective communication of the risks?

"Education" and "general population" both need to be clarified. If education denotes a 30 minute lecture in which a teacher presents information on what HIV/AIDS is, what it does to the infected, how it is transmitted, the statistics of spread, and why not to have risky sex, then in my opinion about 20-30% of the population of India has been "educated". Most of this population is urban. If education means the ability and skills to abstain (or seek gratification in non-penetrative sex) when every cell in the body is focused on sexual gratification through risky sex, or to have the know how and empowerment to use a condom if one is going to have sex outside the one-to-one partner rule, especially when one is under the influence of alcohol and/or drugs, then at most one million people have been educated. (Many times more are relatively "safe" as they are unlikely to have risky sex but even these can be infected by the careless actions of others and exploitation.) Except for some of the very elite schools, most schools do not teach reproductive health or sexuality in any comprehensive way, so even if a lecture on HIV/AIDS is presented, people have little background, training or tools to translate the information into behavior.

In my 4.5 years experience of working with people ranging from elite school and college students to the most conservative and tradition bound villagers, I have not encountered any barriers to education by the public themselves other than, in a few cases, an initial lack of interest. (The barriers I am familiar with are often created by the meeting organizers, political opportunists, religious zealots on the sidelines, or by inadequately informed do-gooders.) The caveat is that you have to first develop trust with the audience. They have to perceive and feel that what you are telling them is correct, that you have come to help them and genuinely care for them, and the message should be delivered without judgment. To be effective, education should be supplemented with counseling. Once a person begins to think about the issues after being presented with information, she/he should have recourse to a counselor (within the family or circle of friends or a professional) to tailor that information to their life and to be able to formulate and take steps that will lead to behavior change or reduce vulnerability. If the latter is the desired level of "education", then it is almost completely missing.

3. How do you think the recent political acknowledgment of the problem will change things for the future? Do you anticipate dramatic decreases in the numbers of people being infected? Or are there barriers that cannot be broken down simply by political will?

By holding of the Parliamentary Forum on the HIV/AIDS, India has taken the first steps and recognized it has a very difficult problem (social, economic, medical, and of national stability) that needs to be confronted with utmost urgency. The country's response so far was summed by Prime Minister A. B. Vajpayee who quoted a wise man as having said "The best time to plant a tree was 20 years ago. The next best time is now." These are indeed wise words. The problem is that the Prime Minister did not "plant the tree" even 20 years later but only talked about planting the tree. The same pattern of action-less talk was then adopted by Shri Manohar Joshi (Lok Sabha Speaker), Smt. Sushma Swaraj (Union Minister of Health and Family Welfare), and Ms. Sonia Gandhi (Leader of the opposition).

No new indigenous funds were allocated for health care or education. All politicians held out their hands to foreign organizations and nations, saying we are ready to act if you give us money. Shri Vajpayee said that "political parties in our country need to pay far greater attention to issues of health care than they do now." Politicians are survival artists with a nose for money, power and publicity. Unfortunately, so far in the fight against HIV/AIDS, most politicians and bureaucrats have appropriated money designated for intervention and the public forum for personal gain and promotion. The speakers did not address the issue of corruption or outline how they were going to change their own behavior. HIV/AIDS is not just a medical problem that a reasonable amount of money (few billion dollars for India) can solve. Its spread also represents a lack of social, medical and economic institutions. The biggest breakdown at the highest level of politics and bureaucracy is self-sacrifice, the concept of nation and society before self and party, and assuming responsibility for the welfare of the public. There was no evidence of a change of behavior in the speakers in this respect or of tangible personal commitment.

Even token but necessary actions were missing. No concession on making treatment a part of the National Policy. No progress on decriminalizing sodomy or prostitution. No statement on the status of development of a curriculum on health and life skills for schools, leave aside its implementation. All the discussion seemed to be on bureaucratic process.

The question "Do you anticipate dramatic decreases in the numbers of people being infected" is hard to quantify since even today surveillance of new infections is poor. My belief is that the actions of the government since 1986, when they first launched the National AIDS Control Program, may have reduced infections by a million people, i.e., there could have been 5.5 million infections if no money from any source, specifically targeted to HIV/AIDS intervention, had been spent. So, to first approximation, the pandemic is following its natural uninterrupted course and the political, bureaucratic, medical, educational and social machinery is still debating and designing road blocks rather than manning established road blocks.

The biggest barrier to be broken down is personal commitment and assuming ownership on part of the politicians, bureaucrats, medical doctors and nurses, and the well-to-do. If past history is an indicator, then the Parliamentary Forum is a necessary first step, but most likely everyone attending or speaking will believe they have done their share for the next year or two. When the numbers jump to 6 million, they will hold the next forum and at that time states which are showing unbelievably low prevalence rates (like Bihar, Jharkhand, Chhatisgarh, and Orissa which have essentially no credible surveillance) will start to appear on the radar screen. My prediction is that adequate social mobilization is unlikely to start before the 10 million HIV+ mark and the government will continue to beg for external funding rather than assume national responsibility. Meanwhile, there is neither a social barrier to limit the spread of HIV nor a barrier to its control if there is political and social will.

4. What is the pattern of spread of HIV/AIDS in India?

The pattern of spread of HIV/AIDS in India is a combination of what is happening in the Western countries and in Sub-Saharan Africa. I illustrate the dominant patterns with the following six examples.

- *Sex-workers:* India's pattern of spread is much closer to Sub-Saharan Africa and South East Asia. Sex-workers are mostly poor, abused both by their pimps and madams and by the police, and without empowerment.
- *Truck Drivers:* Due to their mobility and long hours on the road and away from family, a large fraction of the long haul truck drivers all over the world have risky sexual behavior. They have contributed to the spread of STDs and now HIV/AIDS in the US and in Sub-Saharan Africa. India's pattern is a hybrid of the two.
- *Men having Sex with Men:* India's pattern is common to what is seen throughout South and South-East Asia. Among the well to do it is very similar to the "Down Low" culture of the black and Hispanic MSM community in the USA.
- *IV Drug Use:* People who become addicted to injected drugs are desperate and create a culture of their own. The driver here is access to such drugs. India is sandwiched between the golden triangle (Myanmar, Laos, Northern Thailand, and South China) and the golden triangle (Afghanistan and Pakistan) which together produce 95% of world's heroin, much of which is trafficked through India. In addition, there is a very significant illegal sale of pharmaceutical drugs that is being used as narcotics. Spread of HIV through IV drug use is a much bigger problem than the 'official' claim that it is restricted to the North-Eastern states of Manipur and Nagaland.
- *Migrant Workers:* India's pattern is similar to South Africa's. Industrial and agricultural centers attract workers from all over India, a large fraction of who routinely visit sex-workers. India has over 200 million people who are classified as migrant labor.

- *Vulnerable Children:* This category consists of orphans, abandoned children, child labor and children growing up in abusive homes. According to the UNICEF, there are about 44 million children between the ages of 4-14 that are out of school and doing hazardous work. Many of them are subject to sexual abuse by older men. This trans-generation sexual exploitation puts these children at very high risk for all STDs. This pattern is most similar to that observed in poorer sections of South East Asia and Sub-Saharan Africa.

In a broad sense, the spread amongst the poor is closer to Sub-Saharan Africa model and in the educated and well-to-do it is closer to what is happening in the black and Hispanic communities in the US. Unfortunately, the moralistic stance of India's ultra-conservative politicians, bureaucrats, and religious leaders attempts to lump all these causes into a single widespread belief that moral failure-perceived to be a result of corrupt Western influences-underlies the spread of disease. Unless the true dimension of how prevalent risky sex in all socio-economic strata is and has been prior to even HIV is recognized and accepted, India will not be able to mount an effective HIV/AIDS control.

5. What do you think is missing in the fight against HIV/AIDS in India?

   The biggest shortage today to HIV/AIDS control is not money but caring, committed, knowledgeable people who are willing to work with the marginalized and the poor. One necessary step is to put money directly into organizations that work in a holistic way with the marginalized and the poor, and to develop peer groups. It will be a long time before government agencies are able to work effectively with marginalized and/or high risk populations due to a history of mistrust and the desire to maintain official propriety. Thus NGOs will have to do the bulk of intervention work, so it is important to train and monitor them and help graduate them from doing relief work and/or responding to crises to a holistic portfolio of sustainable development. The government should create laws that allow marginalized and poor communities to have the same human rights as the rest and to hold the law and order organizations responsible for guaranteeing these rights.

The determinants of whether India can control its HIV/AIDS pandemic will be whether there is a comprehensive curriculum on health and life skills that all children can access, the ability of women to negotiate sex safely (as wives, girl friends, or sex workers), whether sodomy and prostitution is decriminalized and corruption is brought under control, and whether children have homes in which they can grow safely with access to health care, education, and nutrition.

## AIDS: Abuses Against Children Rising

Children Affected by HIV/AIDS are facing sustained discrimination and exploitation, finds a new Human Rights Watch report.

July 2004-Anu P., a 6-year-old in Maharashtra, was sent home from kindergarten in 2003 by her teacher. Her grandfather, who had been caring for Anu and her siblings after their parents died of AIDS, explained, "The teacher didn't allow her to come to school because she believes Anu is HIV-positive. I believe that other parents were talking amongst themselves, so the teacher said she shouldn't come." A nearby private doctor told Anu's family not to bring the girl to his clinic "because if you do, other people won't come.'" The reason the man gave, her uncle said, was because of HIV.

Sharmila A., age 10, was HIV-positive and had lost both of her parents to AIDS. She stopped going to school in the fourth grade. "When I went to school, I sat separately from the other children, in the last mat. I sat alone. The other children wanted to be with me, but the teacher would tell them not to play with me. She said, 'This disease will spread to you also, so do not play with her,'" Sharmila said. When she developed tuberculosis, she began traveling some four to five hours to reach a government-run hospital for free medical care. However, the hospital in Tamilnadu did not provide antiretroviral drugs.

and her health did not improve. Sharmila died in January 2004.

These stories and many more are chronicled in a new report "Future Forsaken: Abuses Against Children Affected by HIV/AIDS in India" released yesterday in New Delhi by Human Rights Watch, a New York headquartered NGO. Zama Coursen-Neff, senior researcher with Human Rights Watch's Children's Rights Division is the author. The 209-page report is partly based on her research in India in November and December 2003 and finds that denial and widespread discrimination against children and teenagers are fuelling the already dangerous problem.

In India, most of those dying of AIDS are between fifteen and forty-nine years old, the age when many are raising children. By some estimates, as 1.2 million children under age fifteen in India have lost one or both parents to AIDS. But the number of AIDS orphans has not been adequately or officially measured, All this apart, hundreds of thousands of children are living with HIV/AIDS in India, according to official statistics.

An estimated 2.8 million people died of AIDS in India from 1980 to 2000, and the United Nations (U.N.) projects 12.3 million AIDS deaths from 2000 to 2015.

**Future Forsaken: HRW July 2004:** The Central government has not conducted specific studies to accurately assess the number of children affected by AIDS. "The sixty million dollar question is whether we have accurate data about this problem. This kind of data is simply not being collected", says Zama Coursen-Neff. The general data collected about AIDS patients has not been disaggregated, she adds.

## INFORMATION AND AWARENESS

The report finds that many children-and the professionals who care for them-are not getting the information about HIV they need to protect themselves or to combat discrimination. Even today, fear is rooted in misconceptions that AIDS is a casually transmitted disease. Misinformation and fear is causing some families to reject children who are HIV-positive or who are perceived to be. "There is very low awareness even in government officials. Many teachers, doctors, government officials and ordinary people in India still don't know the basic facts about HIV transmission and AIDS care," says Coursen-Neff.

The report states that fewer than half of all secondary schools offer any AIDS education. Those that do teach about HIV/AIDS do so at an age when most children, especially girls, have already dropped out. And the government is utterly failing to provide information to millions of India's children who are not in school but on the streets, at work, in institutions, in non-formal schools and at home. "But the most vulnerable children are those who've dropped out of school, and they're the ones who are least likely to get lifesaving information about HIV prevention. There are questions about what is being taught, the quality of teaching, and when it is being taught," worries Coursen-Neff.

Although some state governments, like that of Tamilnadu, have begun programs to educate the public, most have not.

## HOW DO CHILDREN CONTRACT AIDS?

India's National AIDS Control Organization (NACO) cites an abundance of routes. The most common route of HIV transmission in India is by sexual transmission and, in the northeast, transmission through injection drug use. Other modes of transmission include blood transfusions and from mother to child during the course of pregnancy, birth, or breastfeeding. Among young children especially, perinatal transmission is the most common source; however, children in India are also acquiring the disease through sexual contact, including sexual abuse; blood transfusions; and unsterilized syringes, including injection drug use. Girls, when subjected to sexual abuse or early marriage or when denied an education, are especially vulnerable.

## NATIONAL AIDS-CONTROL POLICY AND INSTITUTIONS

The National AIDS Control Organization (NACO) is an autonomous body within the Ministry of Health and Family Welfare. It is charged with implementing the government's response to HIV/AIDS prevention and control. It is responsible for providing training, research, surveillance, and program management; collaborating with other ministries and large government-owned enterprises; conducting advocacy; and mobilizing resources.

NACO and the state AIDS control societies' primary activity targeting children has been prevention of mother-to-child transmission, which involves administering a short course of antiretroviral drugs to mother and newborn that greatly reduces the risk of HIV transmission during pregnancy and child birth. They have not implemented programs to address discrimination against HIV/AIDS-affected children in education, health, or other areas, and only a few states, such as Tamilnadu, have funded small projects to care for children living with HIV/AIDS.

The HRW report records NACO's director explanation: "There has been no segment on children in NACO policy per se. Partly the reason is that there is not enough data generated in surveillance specifically on children." According to NACO, U.N. officials, and others, the third phase of the national AIDS program, scheduled to begin in 2004, is likely to contain some provisions for children; however, NACO officials said they could not tell Human Rights Watch what those provisions would be since planning for the third phase had not formally begun at the end of 2003.

## ACKNOWLEDGEMENT OF RISKS

If there is one situation the government has acknowledged, it is that children are a high risk group in the country. HRW documents that citing Crime in India in 1996, the Central Government reported to the Committee on the Rights of the Child, the treaty body that monitors implementation of the Convention on the Rights of the Child, that "the incidence of child rape increased and.... [t]here has also been an increase in the buying of girls for prostitution... and child marriages."

Clearly policy makers and heads of institutions have not connected the dots between their acknowledgement of the risks and the rising reality.

## LACK OF INTEGRATED PAN-ORGANIZATIONAL APPROACH

It isn't that there isn't machinery to respond. The problem seems to be lack of an integrated multi-disciplinary approach to tackle this rising crisis. But this can only come when multiple departments at the Centre and State work together. This is precisely what isn't happening, and children are paying the price, documents the HRW report.

The Ministry of Education and state education departments are responsible for providing free primary education to all children, regardless of their or their care-givers' HIV status. The Department of Women and Children in the Ministry of Human Resource Development develops government policies and legislation for children and women and coordinates other ministries' activities in these areas. It also administers the Integrated Child Development Services (ICDS) program, which includes preschool, and health and nutrition for preschool children, services that are especially important for HIV/AIDS-affected children.

The Ministry of Health and Family Welfare and state-level health departments administer the public health system and medical education. They also oversee NACO and the state AIDS control societies. The Ministry of Health's Department of Family Welfare and its state-level counterparts focus on family planning, and reproductive and child health, both of which should overlap with HIV/AIDS prevention and care for HIV-positive women and children.

The Ministry of Justice and Social Empowerment and corresponding state-level departments are responsible for children in need of care and protection: orphans and neglected children; children out of school, including street children; children in conflict with the law; and other marginalized groups. The Ministry of Labour and state labour departments are responsible for removing children from hazardous and bonded labour, for prosecuting employers, and for rehabilitating the children.

Despite all this, with the exception of a few individuals, most government officials are leaving HIV/AIDS up to NACO and the state AIDS control societies and failing to take responsibility for protecting HIV/AIDS-affected children under their jurisdictions. For example, HRW records in their report that the Secretary of Family Welfare, J. Prasanna Hota said that there was no need to meet with him to discuss his department's policies for HIV/AIDS-affected children because "NACO is heading this." According to Hota, his department was implementing the prevention of mother-to-child transmission program but has no programs or policies of its own for HIV/AIDS-affected children.

One of his state-level counterparts, Tamilnadu Commissioner for Maternal, Child Health and Welfare, who was also the acting Director of Family Welfare, told Human Rights Watch that: As the director of Family Welfare, our primary focus is on controlling the birth rate. We don't directly handle HIV. Even in child welfare we do not handle it. We provide condoms but their main purpose is birth control, not HIV.... We are under the Health Ministry and we take care of the health of the normal child. We don't have anything to do with HIV.... Our aim is a healthy mother, healthy child, and a decrease in the infant and maternal mortality rate.

## THE STATES

State AIDS control societies, with funds and technical and policy guidance from NACO, are responsible for implementing the National AIDS Prevention and Control Policy. The state AIDS control societies are supposed to contract with NGOs to implement blood safety programs, interventions with high-risk populations, educational campaigns, voluntary counseling and testing, and care and support of people living with HIV/AIDS.

But while state AIDS control societies exist in every state and in certain municipalities, their effectiveness reportedly varies widely. According to the World Bank in 2003, one-third of the posts in all state AIDS control societies remained unfilled, as was the case in 1995; many NGOs lacked the technical capacity to implement national policies; interventions were still very few for "high risk" men other than truckers; and NACO was failing to provide sufficient technical assistance to state AIDS control societies, many of which, in turn, were not providing sufficient supervision or technical assistance to NGOs delivering services.

## GOING FORWARD

Even without the AIDS crisis, the public education and health systems in the country are in a broken situation. When delivery of elementary education and health care are poorly managed, starved of funds and plainly aren't working, why does Coursen-Neff think that these systems must be able to handle a crisis or an impending crisis like this one?

Coursen-Neff admits that delivery of basic services is a huge problem in India and the system simply isn't coping. "But this doesn't address the discrimination aspect—governments have to ensure that children aren't turned away from schools and facilities. Monitoring for discrimination has to be a key component. Doctors, training academies, care-givers, government officials all have to part of a newer awareness and anti-discrimination strategy", she points out.

In sum, the HRW report warns that the rising incidence of HIV/AIDS and the risk of HIV/AIDS in children is simply not on the radar screen of public health institutions. Second, discrimination against infected children and un-infected children of infected relatives/adult parents remains and this is likely to exacerbate the problem. And all of this will only further undermine the national anti-AIDS policy and put millions of lives at risk. Human Rights Watch has called on the Indian government to take immediate action to enact and enforce legislation proscribing discrimination against people living with HIV/AIDS; include for teeth in legislation so that children may never be barred from school solely because they are HIV-positive; ensure that children living with HIV/AIDS receive all available medical care, including antiretroviral treatment; provide all children, both in and out of school, with comprehensive, accurate and age-appropriate information about HIV/AIDS.

## HIV/AIDS IS KILLING INNOCENT WOMEN AND GIRLS

Today is World AIDS Day, a day of remembrance for the over 20 million people worldwide who have died from this disease and the tens of millions suffering from it today. The people of the United States join with the people of India in mourning the lives that have been lost to HIV/AIDS.

HIV/AIDS is the most serious public health challenge facing India today. India is at a critical juncture in the epidemic. While millions are already infected, it is estimated that last year 500,000 more Indians contracted the virus. We still can contain this epidemic, and I am pleased to re-affirm America's support to India in combating the scourge of this disease.

The theme for World AIDS Day this year is "Women, Girls and HIV/AIDS." In India 36% of the people estimated to be living with HIV are women, and the potential for a much higher number is real. In sub-Saharan Africa, the proportion is 57 percent. Young girls are particularly vulnerable, in some African communities, as many as 20 percent of girls aged 15-19 are infected, compared to just 5 percent of boys the same age. Worldwide, almost 50 percent of HIV-positive people are women.

HIV is spreading rapidly among females for many reasons. The lower status of women and girls and practices such as male infidelity, prostitution, child sexual abuse, and sex trafficking are important factors. In addition, male-to-female HIV transmission during sex is about twice as likely to occur as female-to-male transmission.

In India, awareness of HIV/AIDS among women is also distressingly low—only 20 percent of women in some areas have correct knowledge about the disease. Women are less likely to access care and treatment and are often subject to severe stigma and discrimination, even within their own families. Reports also indicate that the rate of female injecting drug use, another common way HIV/AIDS is transmitted, is increasing.

Even when they are not themselves infected, women are victimized by HIV/AIDS in other ways. They are essential caretakers, caring for the sick and raising orphaned children. They also suffer from stigma and rejection by family and neighbors.

Mary, a 30-year-old woman living near Chennai, provides a powerful story of hope. Her husband abruptly abandoned her, pregnant, after learning she was HIV positive. When she went into labor she was refused treatment by one hospital and referred to another. Fearing a second rejection, she returned home, only to give birth en route. Her neighbors, when they learned she had been refused from a hospital, asked her to vacate her house, at which point her mother contacted the NGO Community Health Education Society (CHES) for help.

CHES provided immediate basic medical advise, but more importantly worked extensively with her neighbors to show them she was not a threat. CHES staff spent time with Mary and the baby, kissed the child publicly and drank water from Mary's house. They visited her regularly and now notice she receives open support from her neighbors.

While U.S.-India relations have never been better—some say they are at "an all time high"-we must work doubly hard in the fight against HIV/AIDS. I believe the breadth and depth of our joint efforts against HIV/AIDS exemplify the transforming nature of our relationship-but we need more.

The U.S. Government dedicates $33 million annually to fighting HIV/AIDS in India. The United States Agency for International Development (USAID) and the Centers for Disease Control and Prevention (CDC) spend $18 million on HIV/AIDS-related programs and the National Institutes of Health (NIH) invests $15 million on U.S.-India biomedical and public health research on the disease. In addition, the United States is the single largest donor country to the Global AIDS Fund to Fight HIV, TB, and Malaria.

U.S. non-governmental organizations also play an important role. The Bill and Melinda Gates Foundation, the Bill Clinton Foundation, the Richard Gere Foundation, and the Elizabeth Glaser Pediatric AIDS Foundation are also active here. These public and private partnerships share knowledge, technology, research and resources that bring our countries closer together.

And corporations are taking leadership roles as well, with companies such as the Ford, General Electric, Dell, Bharat Petroleum and TATA actively fighting HIV/AIDS, trafficking in women, and other issues related to the disease.

U.S. Government programs focus on preventing new infections, bringing lifesaving treatment to people with HIV, and caring for those infected and affected by the disease, including orphans and vulnerable children. Scientists from India and the United States are working together on the development of vaccines and microbicides for HIV/AIDS. Their combined efforts may one day lead to the development of a safe and effective vaccine that we desperately need to fight this disease.

We are also partnering with the Government of India, NGOs and the private sector to combat the commercial sexual exploitation of women and children, child sexual abuse and rape. In the past five years, the USG has invested $1.8 million to fund 34 Indian NGOs working on issues related to child sexual abuse and trafficking in women and children. These projects are spread throughout India and address the full range of prevention, arrest, protection, prosecution and rehabilitation issues related to trafficking victims. For example, the U.S. Government funded one of India's most effective anti-trafficking organizations, STOP-helping it rescue 450 victims of forced prostitution that lead to the arrest of 155 traffickers and 68 trafficker convictions in 2004 alone.

Protecting women and girls, like the fight against HIV/AIDS generally, is an effort in which everyone has a part to play. The American people are privileged to join the people of India as we work together to turn the tide against HIV/AIDS

The spread of HIV/AIDS depends on, and exposes, every weakness in society. It spreads if there is poverty, illiteracy, lack of public health, if women do not have reproductive rights, if the use of alcohol and narcotics is high and widespread, and if corruption becomes part of daily life. The last, corruption, also precludes the possibility of adequate response by the government or the bureaucracy. It is for these reasons that HIV/AIDS is not simply a medical disease but also a social one. In this article I would like to bring to light some less frequently discussed behaviors, social patterns, and practices that are fueling the spread of sexually transmitted diseases, of which Hepatitis B and C, and HIV/AIDS are devastating to the individual and the society. I will also discuss two very different examples of successful intervention and recent developments in treatment that provide a glimmer of hope in the global fight against HIV/AIDS.

India has a very large migrant work force, both industrial and agricultural, estimated at over 200 million, and increasing in numbers due to the growing population. Furthermore, every natural disaster (Orissa cyclone, Rajasthan drought, Bhuj earthquake) displaces people and adds to the ranks of the migrants. A majority of those on the move are men who work under harsh conditions to save as much as possible for their families. Their life styles and conditions expose them to alcohol and drug addiction and to risky sex. They return home sporadically, often carrying diseases to their spouses. This migrant labor force is very often served by a community of sex workers, that is itself migrant and indistinguishable; many cities do not have well-defined "red-light" areas which serve as focal points for sex work. Reaching these sex workers is, therefore, hard; their education and empowerment remains at the same level as that of the work force at large.

It is an open secret that Karol Bagh area in New Delhi is the focal point for sex workers from Russia and eastern Europe. (Other metropolitan cities also have their analogue areas and risk populations, like trips to Thailand, call-girls, college students, etc.). I have often heard mentioned the thrill of a joust with blue-eyed, blond, sex goddesses; people are clearly oblivious of the high rates of prevalence of Hepatitis and HIV in this group, or are willing to take the risk. The pattern of operation of these sex workers is that they smuggle goods into India, work as high class call girls while in India, and then smuggle Indian goods and narcotics when going back. One can only wonder who their clients are since their evening charges are higher than the monthly salary of 99 percent of Indians. Unfortunately, lack of political will and corruption is preventing adequate intervention.

India is sandwiched between the two major heroin producing areas of the world—the golden triangle (Myanmar, Laos, Thailand) and the golden crescent (Afganistan and Pakistan)—which account for roughly 95 percent of the world's heroin. India itself produces significant quantities of opium, hashish, and ganja. Historically, the use of these narcotics has been a part of the life of rural Indians, blue collared workers, and urban slum dwellers. They have used it as part of evening entertainment, relaxation, and community activities. What is different today is the amount, variety, and toxicity of drugs available. For example, opium use is a widespread and huge problem in the districts of Punjab bordering Pakistan, and in Rajasthan west of Jodhpur. The concentration of narcotics in chewing tobacco and "gutka" is growing, and the number of people using them throughout the day is also growing. Intravenous use of heroin has already resulted in an HIV crises in Mizoram, Manipur, and Nagaland. There is growing incidence of IV heroin use (and of other opiates, tranquilizers, and sedatives that are easily available from many pharmacists) amongst school and college students in all major cities and, we see, widespread in Punjab, Haryana, and Rajasthan. This growing threat of drugs is, in itself, a nightmare for the nation and needs a major intervention program, but coupled with HIV it will be devastating as demonstrated by the experience in Mizoram, Manipur, and Nagaland. The authorities are aware of the severity of the problem in the border states, however, lack of political will and corruption has, and is, preventing adequate response to the widespread drug problem.

In the affluent classes evening entertainment is synonymous with hours of intensive drinking. The quality and quantity of single malt scotch consumed has become a status symbol. It should, therefore, come as no surprise that younger and younger children are imitating their parents and elders, and for them risky behavior includes alcohol, drugs, and sex. (A very high correlation has been observed between these three risky behaviors). These children are often left without responsible supervision and with ample funds for days at end and while the parents are on business trips. Sexual experimentation, with HIV ever waiting, is proving deadly for many. Alcohol use amongst the poor has reached nightmarish proportions; the government, mindful only of the welcome increase in taxes collected, is seemingly oblivious of the eventual cost to the society and the nation.

The increasing reliance on television, alcohol, and gambling as the most common outlets for stress and tensions, and the predominant form of entertainment is a devastating social behavior with far reaching consequences. For example, it has become an underlying cause of risky sexual behavior. To counter this "way of life" requires development of alternate forms of entertainment, and the awareness on why the constructive use of leisure time is a necessary life-long habit (life-skill) that needs to be developed early in life. (Possible activities include voluntary community improvement programs, spending more time with children, reading, sports and other outdoor activities). Facilitating such a change in life-style is a Herculean task considering that a significant fraction of a society of 1 billion has already become addicted to television and alcohol. The problem of drug addiction, however, will only become worse if people do not develop such life-skills.

It has become amply clear that in India's middle and upper classes, the onset of sexual experimentation and development of risky sexual behavior is occurring in mid-to-late teens. The most vulnerable time being the transition from school to college, especially amongst boys and girls from rural backgrounds going to colleges in cities. Consequently, awareness and intervention programs have to begin in schools and before risky behaviors become addictive habits. In my experience, schools are very open to providing awareness, but are relying on external speakers since their staff is reluctant and/or un-prepared to speak on relevant issues of sexuality and sex. Thus, the exposure is sporadic, hurried, and inadequate; only a fraction of the senior classes attend a given session and the information is expected to trickle down to the rest, or they must wait for the next speaker who may come months or years later.

This is true even in the very elite schools of India which have English as the medium of instruction; a language that possesses a clinical vocabulary on sex. In most Indian languages the lack of such a vocabulary has attached a perception of vulgarity to discussions of sexuality, reproductive health, methods of birth control, and sexually transmitted diseases. As a result most students ( well over 90 percent of the total students in India, and all those not able to go to school) still do not get adequate information from reliable sources—parents, trained teachers, or counselors.

On the treatment front there is very good news. The year 2001 has already provided the world with two miraculous gifts, whose resonant application can start to make a difference immediately. First, is the growing widespread acceptance of the Brazilian experiment—providing Highly Aggressive Anti-Retroviral Therapy (HAART) to all HIV/AIDS patients. This has resulted, in Brazil, in holding down the rate of new infections at the 1995 level, and given a life to those infected. (A summary of the Brazil experiment can be obtained from the New York Times). The second is the bold offer by the Indian Pharmaceutical manufacturer CIPLA to provide the cocktail drugs (three drugs including reverse transcriptase and protease inhibitors) at cost (\$1200 to wholesalers, \$600 to Governments, and \$350 to non-profit charitable organizations like Medicines Sans Frontieres). Details of the CIPLA offer can be obtained at CIPLA OFFER.

The above two breakthroughs, while being landmarks and essential in the fight against the spread of HIV/AIDS, are, by themselves, not enough. For example, most of the estimated four million Indians infected with HIV are not aware of their status. In fact, only a few percent are. So, in view of the long term solution, having HAART available is not very helpful unless we have the capacity to prevent infections or, if they happen, to intervene very early. Given the non-specific symptoms of HIV infection in early stages, which may last years, there is no motivation for the masses to seek the specific blood test unless the awareness levels are very high.

Today, most HIV infections are being detected at very late stages when serious opportunistic infections force the poor and the marginalized to seek medical help. Diagnosis late in the progression of the disease has two disastrous consequences. First, the continued risky behaviors during the time of the undetected infection put others at risk, and second, since HAART does not undo the damage to the body and the immune system already caused by the virus (HAART significantly reduces further degeneration by reducing the viral load to negligible amounts and hence the transmission rate), late detection means living with a highly compromised system even if HAART was made available.

Even with CIPLA's offer there are still remain problems of implementation for which there seems to be no political will.

At $350 per year, the cost to Indian Government to treat the roughly 4 million infected would be over two billion dollars per year once delivery and test costs are included. This amount is roughly eight times the FY2001 yearly budget of the Ministry of Health, Central government. As a result, I do not foresee the Indian government acting on the CIPLA offer in the near future unless the price drops by another factor of ten. Their concern may be that if they provide free drugs for HIV, then they will have to provide free drugs for all life-threatening communicable diseases. My contention is that they should and must provide drugs for all serious communicable diseases and make health a national priority. Those in power need to study the Brazilian experiment, and if nothing else, read the New York times article mentioned above. Lack of action by India, to my mind, is a clear example of a short sighted policy since, today, a very effective program can be started for a much smaller amount as only 3-4 percent of the estimated infections have been diagnosed.

Today, there is much debate whether India has the infrastructure in place to administer HAART. In my opinion the answer is clear and simple—we need to start providing the drugs today even if the necessary infrastructure needs development. Today, the majority of doctors are decoupled and disengaged from the HIV/AIDS crises because they feel powerless—there is nothing they can do to help the infected. Making drugs available to them to administer will lead to their becoming engaged, learning about the disease, and thus providing the infrastructure that is arguably missing today. It will also go a long way in removing the stigma associated with the disease, give a life to those infected, and allow many of the HIV+ to become peer educators.

There is good news on the vaccine development front also. After years of pessimism and setbacks, the new influx of money from government and non-government sources has created a number of very large and international collaborations who are investigating/developing/using innovative techniques for making vaccines. While there are many new developments, new ideas, promising directions, and candidate vaccines, the fact remains that there is no vaccine at this point of time. Also, unless the vaccine has very high efficacy (over 80 percent), awareness leading to behavior changes will continue to be essential. I feel that it is essential to proceed by emphasising prevention under the assumption that there will be no vaccine for the next ten years at least.

Societal response to build the capacity to spread awareness, to provide HIV testing, pre-and post-test counseling, and to improve the monitoring of blood in blood banks, is slowly gaining momentum. For the purposes of illustration I will discuss two very different examples of social intervention on health that I am familiar with. During my recent visit to India, I had the good fortune to interact with Arpana Research and Charities Trust near Karnal in Haryana, and Association Francois-Xavier Bagnoud (FXB) in India.

Arpana Trust is a charitable hospital, and a village outreach program. It is part of a religious organization (Ma's ashram) and draws its inspiration from it. Over the last twenty years it has built an excellent reputation amongst the surrounding communities, and now provides health care in 35 surrounding villages. Its main medical facility specializes in maternal issues and in eye care. It is equipped with the latest technology and staffed by enviable doctors. The institution is so unique that I was prompted to ask the Director, Dr Ela Anand, why the lines of people waiting for care, seen at all hospitals, were not present.

The reason, she said with a smile, is that we have a very strong village outreach program and most of the day to day issues are taken care of at that level and early so that many serious complications do not develop. She then went on to explain how they have involved the villagers in water management programs; never providing anything for free but always making villagers partners. The most difficult program, which the staff is also the most proud of, has been the payback of microloans given to women, and their success in training the village women to manage money and learn to trust and use banks to accumulate savings. My final question to her, in order to understand risk factors for HIV, was—what is the incidence of sexually transmitted diseases (STD)? At this she shook her head and said that the village women do not come to them for

STD treatment—their sense of shame is too great. They go to quacks and so called venereal disease specialists where they feel anonymous, or suffer PID in silence. What the hospital is seeing increasing numbers of are young women coming in for treatment for sterility. She suspects that the underlying cause, in most cases, is STDs, but due to ignorance and sense of shame the women come to the hospital too late for her to reverse the problem. This experience of Arpana is a clear statement that progress in female reproductive health and their empowerment to avoid STDs is perhaps the most significant indicator of human development.

FXB India is a non-profit organization with headquarters in Switzerland and who now have a major effort in India. They started work on HIV in Rajasthan in June, 2000. In this short time they already have a functioning testing and counseling center in Sumerpur in Rajasthan, an outreach program, have developed a collaboration with the blood banks including the zonal blood bank at Umaid hospital in Jodhpur, and are now rapidly duplicating this success across India. The novelty of their approach is to build capacity rapidly by identifying "leaders" all over India and empowering them to build a program similar to their Rajasthan experiment, rather than waiting to refine every detail.

To supplement the local expertise, they are inviting an international team of experts to provide the latest training in counseling, evaluation, and capacity building. The program is being developed with the clear realization that the infrastructure has to be robust and resilient enough to last the two-three decades that such programs will have to be in place to combat HIV even if a cure, or less than 100 percent effective vaccine, is found in the next ten years. There is no doubt that such a program requires significant funding, however, society as a whole has to accept the need, and bear the responsibility for, generating this if they wish to get rid of the scourge of HIV/AIDS.

I believe that having such different organizations like Arpana and FXB India, and the whole range in between, is healthy and essential. What is also essential is to develop a network linking them so that experiences can be documented, shared, and evaluated. We have much to learn from each other and the time is short.

There are many other excellent organizations working hard to stop the spread of HIV/AIDS and raise social awareness. However, it would be naive to assume that India has finally developed the infrastructure to deal with the crisis. My feeling is that we are just finally beginning. The efforts of organizations dedicated to HIV intervention, like FXB India, need to grow by at least two to three orders of magnitude and become far more cohesive.

The task of dealing with societal issues and the consequent risk for HIV/AIDS is Herculean and overwhelming. Today, adequate intervention requires mobilization of a significant part of society. Many more caring people must join the fight and be empowered by a much larger budget, both from the government and from private individuals and corporations. With current levels of effort, the HIV infections will still continue to grow. There is optimism provided by the recent developments, but this optimism will prove disastrous if it leads to complacency

## HIV/AIDS DATA

At the end of 1999 it was estimated that there were a total of 3,700,000 adults and children living with HIV in India, of whom 3,500,000 were adults (including 1,300,000 women and 160,000 children). During 1999 there were thought to be 310,000 HIV related deaths. It is estimated also that at the end of 1999 there a total of 557,570 children under the age of 15 were orphaned through the loss of mothers or both parents to HIV/AIDS.

According to the UNAIDS epidemiological fact sheet for India: "Scattered surveillance studies have been conducted in India since the late 1980's. It was not until 1998 that the National AIDS Control Organization made a concerted attempt to conduct consistent HIV surveillance in each state.

The available results show that HIV prevalence among antenatal clinic women tested in the major urban centers of Calcutta, Mumbai and New Delhi, median HIV prevalence has increased from 0 percent in the late 1980s to 2 percent in 1999.

In Mumbai, the major urban area in western India, HIV prevalence has increased from 1 percent in 1993 to 3 percent in 1999. Outside of the major urban areas, median HIV prevalence among antenatal women tested in 1999 was 0.3 percent. HIV prevalence was 0 percent in 34 of the 86 reporting sites.

Among sex workers tested in Mumbai, HIV prevalence had reached 51 percent in 1993. In Calcutta, 12 percent of sex workers tested in 1997 were HIV positive. In 1999, 58 percent of sex workers tested in Vellore and 11 percent of sex workers tested in Agra were HIV positive. In 1998 and 1999, HIV testing among STD clinic patients became part of the National AIDS Control Organization sentinel surveillance system. In 1999, 4 percent of STD clinic patients tested in the major urban areas were HIV positive, however the range was from 1 percent in New Delhi to 64 percent in Mumbai. Outside of the major urban areas, a median of 2 percent of STD patients tested at 71 sentinel sites were HIV positive with a range of 0 to 45 percent. HIV prevalence among IV drug users in Manipur State increased from 9 percent in 1989 to 85 percent in 1993. In 1999, 68 percent of IV drug users in Churachandpur and 49 percent of IV drug users in Imphal tested HIV positive. In 1995, HIV testing of truck drivers at 9 sites found 2 percent of drivers HIV positive. In 1996, 6 percent of truck drivers tested in Namakkal and 5 percent tested in Tiruchirapalli were HIV positive. In Salem, 1 percent of truck drivers tested between 1994 and 1997 were HIV positive.

On a local scale, in different parts of the country, community based responses are addressing the epidemic with some degree of success. Among the most notable of these is the Sonagachi project in the state of West Bengal. This has led not only to a reduction in HIV prevalence among sex workers, but it has contributed to increased self-esteem, better organisation and a sense of agency among local communities.

## BRIEF DESCRIPTION

Supporting community responses has been a significant feature of the UNDP response to the HIV epidemic at both global and national levels. A key component of this has been the development of strategic partnerships with civil society organisations which have the potential to play critical roles in the national response. This includes not only those groups and organisations which work exclusively on HIV/AIDS issues but also those which are involved in development more generally. UNDP has been especially eager to support the greater involvement of the latter group because of their sheer number in India and more importantly because their work links so clearly to the socio-economic determinants of the epidemic.

In some countries initial responses to the HIV epidemic have relied upon the assumptions that the fundamental problem to be addressed is one of lack of knowledge and that, in itself, the provision of information will lead to behaviour change. Hence, drawing upon experience of other health and development issues such as population and reproductive health, water and sanitation, countries have invested in large-scale IEC campaigns, sometimes in combination with more focused educational programmes for specific ""susceptible" groups. However, the large-scale nature of these activities tend to result in content which is general rather than specific, simple rather than complex, and externally determined rather than locally generated.

Not surprisingly, impact evaluation consistently reveals significant potential in terms of creating changes in awareness but much less convincing evidence to demonstrate impact upon behaviour. One broad conclusion from this experience is that awareness is a necessary, but rarely sufficient, step in the process towards behaviour change. Another broad conclusion is that risk-associated behaviours such as unprotected sexual intercourse (which accounts for the vast majority of HIV infections in India), or sharing of equipment among injecting drug users, are fundamentally social events, involving more than one person and occurring within specific social, cultural and economic settings.

Thus, it was felt that the focus of programmes might need to shift from the level of the 'individual' to that of 'the community'. In many communities throughout India the most credible sources of support are the numerous NGOs involved in a vast array of local health and development issues.

Furthermore, in many countries, and particularly in India, there already exists a considerable accumulation of expertise in relation to participatory development. This approach is based upon fundamental principles of locally determined problem solving based on respect for local knowledge and values.

It was in recognition of the above that UNDP decided to support a pilot initiative in order to identify and demonstrate ways of generating relevant and sustainable local responses to the epidemic by building upon local expertise and partnership across traditional sectoral boundaries.

**Goal**

The project goal and objectives were as follows:

- To stimulate processes of learning among development and HIV/AIDS practitioners, and among NGO, private and government sectors in India.
- To increase the capacity of development NGOs in India to respond to some of the developmental dimensions of HIV/AIDS in ways which are participatory and consistent with good practice in relation to HIV/AIDS.

And more specifically:

- To enhance understanding about the social and economic causes and consequences of the epidemic;
- To promote more effective community based responses to strengthen government and NGO partnerships at the state and district levels;
- To expand collaboration between various development partners to jointly address the challenges posed by the epidemic.

**Brief History**

Building upon a history of activities in India relating to HIV and Development, including support for a situational and needs analysis of NGOs in 1995, a consultant visited a number of NGOs during 1996/7 in order to explore the learning approaches currently used by these organisations. The consultant noted the wealth of experience among the NGOs in terms of work on HIV/AIDS issues but also highlighted the potential constraint imposed by a preponderance of "message-oriented" approaches (IEC). The limitations of this approach to HIV/AIDS were indicated: for example it is unlikely that a narrow focus on behaviour, without appropriate consideration of context and the human relationships within which such behaviour occurs, will necessarily lead to behaviour change. Some NGOs, which had already used such approaches, expressed frustration that they had been unable to achieve the goal of behaviour change which they had set for their work. It was noted that additional efforts were needed to enhance understanding and skills in relation to the application of participatory approaches.

On the basis of these broad findings, UNDP organised an Informal Consultation (Delhi, 18-20 February 1998). The goals of the Consultation were to bring together a number of NGOs in order to share experiences of working on HIV/AIDS issues, particularly in relation to the learning methodologies and tools employed in this work, and to explore the development of collaborative local strategies for expanding the use of participatory approaches to learning in relation to HIV/AIDS issues. Participants were primarily those involved in training and communication and represented NGOs from Chennai, Mumbai, Pune and Delhi.

The Consultation provided participants with the opportunity to experience a range of evocative participatory tools designed specifically to address HIV/AIDS issues within a broad context of social and economic development. These activities provided an opportunity for participants to clarify differences between message-oriented IEC approaches and participatory approaches which are experiential, interactive and dynamic, and which engage people as equal partners in defining their own problems and solutions.

The meeting also highlighted a number of challenges posed by the need for more effective networking and capacity development among NGOs and for greater cooperation between NGOs and government. Moreover the issues raised during the consultation were supportive of national efforts to promote more effective community-based initiatives and to enhance government/NGO collaboration as reflected in the national strategy.

Towards the end of the Consultation, participants developed follow-up strategies for strengthening their own capacity in relation to the development, implementation and evaluation of participatory approaches, and for sharing the experience and outcomes of the Consultation with other NGOs in their local areas.

UNDP provided participants with training on HIV and development and followed this with seed funding for each participating state to conduct its own capacity building event on HIV and Development, where necessary drawing upon the technical resources available within the 'core' group. In this way the number of advocates of participatory approaches to learning about HIV was increased in a number of states. The project culminated in a training of trainers on HIV and which took place in December 1998.

## MAJOR ELEMENTS OF THE PROJECT

### Drawing on Existing Resources

Along with many other organisations, UNDP has a long history of involvement in participatory approaches to development issues. It was felt that this experience and accumulated expertise might prove to be of considerable value in providing assistance to a range of NGOs which expressed interest in developing the nature and impact of their educational/ communications work. To this end, a consultant with several decades' experience of participatory methodologies was recruited to undertake needs assessment activities, to develop a number of pilot participatory tools relevant to developmental aspects of HIV/AIDS and to write these up in the form of a toolkit. Similar sharing of experiences was also made possible through participation of a consultant with many years experience in West Africa. Finally, and most important in terms of sharing of experience, was the involvement of a strong, vocal group of individuals with many years experience between them in terms of working on HIV/AIDS. In contrast to many similar meetings, the vast majority of participants and facilitators were of Indian origin, looking inwards among peers for strategies and solutions instead of depending upon 'outsiders' to define the problem and determine the solutions. Explicitly, the process drew upon an existing pool of competent trainers within the country, and focused upon enhancing their capacity to respond to the emerging challenges posed by the epidemic in India. Through a number of local situation assessments, together the knowledge and expertise of the group members, the process could be adapted as necessary to respond to a richer understanding of local realities of HIV/AIDS in India, building drawing upon local knowledge and expertise instead of the assumptions which so often guide development initiatives.

### Situation Assessments

The history of this project dates back to 1995 when UNDP provided support for a situational assessment and needs analysis of NGOs in India in relation to the epidemic. The report drew attention to the need for increasing partnership between government and NGOs as well as the need for capacity development building among NGOs. Subsequently a consultant visited a number of NGOs during 1996 and 1997 and drew attention to the specific need for enhanced understanding and skills in the use of participatory approaches in relation to HIV/AIDS which would be both more consistent with the community focus of these organisations and more relevant to generating the kinds of solutions to the epidemic which would be locally relevant and sustainable. Participatory Research in Asia were commissioned to undertake an analysis of organizations currently using participatory approaches.

### Training in HIV and Development

The Informal Consulation led to UNDP support for a training workshop (July 1998) which was provided for NGO representatives on HIV and Development. Similar workshops were then implemented in seven States with financial support from UNDP and technical support provided as necessary by more experienced NGOs. A Training of Trainers workshop was held in December 1998 (with a preparatory meeting held in New Delhi in September 1998) and included a number of participants from the state level workshops.

## Gender Dimensions

As elsewhere the HIV epidemic in India is a gendered phenomenon, affecting women and men, boys and girls, in different ways which reflect their social, cultural and economic status. For this reason, among others, gender considerations were an integral aspect of the project and reflected in a number of ways: for example:

- the selection of individuals and organisations participating in project events and workshops;
- a set of learning tools, designed specifically for the Indian context, with the purpose of enhancing understanding of the gender dimensions of the causes and consequences of the HIV epidemic;
- broad representation with the planning group of a number of organisations that involved in advocacy work on gender and development concerns.

## Core Planning Group

Over the course of the project, a local core planning group gradually came together and begun to assume ownership from UNDP for the project at national level. A planning meeting was organised in October 1998 where this group was more formally established and where it assumed responsibility for a number of concrete project activities.

## Documentation

As a pilot project which is designed to address development issues, documentation of this initiative has been an important element of the project, not only in terms of recording the project's "institutional memory", but also in terms of generating and disseminating broader lessons learned.

Documentation produced by the project was developed in response to the specific felt needs of participants who expressed a wish for material which captured the "life of the process" and which made available to others the learning resulting from the project. In addition to consultancy reports and project updates, the following documents have been produced:

- Support to the Future Role of NGOs in HIV and Development in India (1997)
- Report of an Informal Consultation: Strengthening Community-Based Responses to HIV/AIDS (1998)
- Participatory Toolkit for Strengthening Community Responses to HIV/AIDS (2000)

## Partnerships and Alliances

The concepts of partnership and alliance have been placed at the centre of this project. The project itself was evidence of partnership between UNDP (both the global HIV and Development Programme (HDP) and the field office) and UNAIDS (and other UN agencies including UNIFEM). Partnerships were established at all levels: national, state and local, and across sectors and disciplines. At certain levels (for example the core NGO group), the partnerships have gone on to have an independent existence beyond the project.

The conceptual framework of the project highlights the importance of ongoing policy dialogue (for example with between HDP and the UNDP Field Office, with UNAIDS and with NACO) in establishing a sufficiently enabling environment within which the project could be implemented. Strategic linkages with key stakeholders were established and reinforced on a regular basis. Attention was paid to clarifying the possible roles which might be played by NACO in this process, a key variable given NACO's pivotal role in facilitating collaboration and partnership at national level and in setting an example for state level coordination and activity.

## Monitoring and Evaluation

The project was closely monitored by through periodic visits, submission of reports and via regular telephone and email communication between UNDP (New York) and the field office in India, and within India among UNDP, UNAIDS, NACO and the NGOs.

Preliminary discussion on evaluation within the project highlighted the distinction between evaluation of the individual components of the project (for example the training workshops) and of the process and outcomes of the project itself. An important component of the evaluation has consisted in the consolidation of the project documentation with a focus on identification of lessons learned. Another important aspect was the production of an autonomous evaluation report by one of the project participants.

At the level of outputs, the project has delivered in a number areas: selection criteria were established for the selection of NGOs to participate in the capacity-building activities; capacity has been developed among a broad range of NGOs, private and governmental institutions from different regions of India and a body of documentation produced which describes the process and unfolding of the project.

In terms of outcomes, it is inevitably more difficult to state these with confidence. Nonetheless it is clear that the consistent focus upon a transparent and participatory process (mirroring the content of the project) allowed a group of key individuals to establish themselves as a group which became committed to addressing developmental dimensions of HIV/AIDS in participatory ways. This commitment was reflected in the professional and proficient way in which they undertook capacity building work within their own states before coming together again to design, organise and facilitate a successful HIV and development workshop.

Awareness has been increased among participating groups, both of the development implications of the epidemic and of the place of participatory approaches within community responses. A gendered approach has been adopted within the project from the outset and has included the use of a training module on gender, development and the HIV epidemic.

The group, brokered by UNDP, established a process of dialogue with NACO, something which had previously proved problematic. This however seems not to have lasted, and suggests the potential value of an 'honest broker' role filled by someone who is trusted by both parties and perceived not to be pursuing their own political agenda.

Individual components of the project were each evaluated. Since the project focused largely upon capacity development through training, participant evaluation sheets formed the bulk of the data for this. The formal publication resulting from the project the 'Toolkit' has only just become available and its impact, therefore impossible to assess. Nonetheless, some of the activities have been incorporated within the UNDP HIV and Development Workshop materials and used with great success in the Caribbean and Central America.

**Results to Date:**

- Documentation of the capacity of, and learning approaches used by, NGOs in India.
- A set of participatory learning tools designed and tested specifically to raise and explore some of the development implications of the epidemic.
- Establishment of a core group of NGO representatives (from both HIV/AIDS and development sectors) as advocates of the need to address developmental causes and consequences of the HIV epidemic and of the use of participatory approaches in mobilising community responses to it.
- Collaborative mechanisms identified with UNAIDS (co-sponsors and secretariat) and NACO.

**The Future**

Towards the end of the project, action plans were prepared by participants from six different states and local funding secured (and administered through the UNDP country office) for their operationalisation. These plans are currently in the process of implementation.

Lessons learned through this project are being widely shared, not only within India and the Asia region but beyond. For example the toolkit has been shared with all UNDP country offices and will also be available in French and Spanish.

**Best Practice**

Lessons Learned:

- The NGO sector in India is a vital (and often untapped) resource in addressing the development dimensions of the HIV epidemic, but within the sector there is considerable variation in terms of existing capacity.

- Consistent, careful attention to process is critical if initiatives are to become locally owned and sustainable.
- External agencies can act in the role of catalyst, advocate, mobiliser of resources and honest broker among stakeholders, particularly when such dialogue is rare or absent.
- Considerable capacity already exists within the NGO sector-HIV/AIDS specific and general development NGOs can both teach and learn from each other.
- Networks which emerge in response to locally determined processes are ultimately likely to be more sustainable and effective than those which are artificially created by external agencies.
- Considerably increased impact can be achieved through a strategic approach to capacity development.
- This in turn, requires that NGO efforts be firmly located within the contexts of ongoing national, state level and local activities.
- A methodical, systematic approach to capacity development which builds upon existing strengths can engage and significantly strengthen the response to the development challenges to the NGO sector.
- Tensions between government and NGOs are inevitable, and brokering by a third party can at times be necessary and useful. Conflict need not necessarily be destructive. The ongoing, periodic tensions between the project partner NGOs and government, demonstrate that the project did not end with the funding: it is vibrantly alive

## The Setting

India, a country of over 1 billion people, is the world's largest democracy. Located in the South Asian region, this sub-continent shares political borders with Pakistan and Afghanistan in the West and Bangladesh and Myanmar in the East. In the South, India is separated from Sri Lanka by a narrow channel of Indian Ocean. The second largest populous country of the world is administratively divided in 29 States and 6 Union Territories. India has 18 officially recognized languages including English.

In India the first case of HIV was reported in 1986 in Chennai (then Madras). Since then the presence of the virus has been reported from all parts of the country. The National AIDS Control Organization of India (NACO) has established HIV/AIDS surveillance in all the states of the country. All information pertaining to HIV/AIDS are primarily based on the reports received from these surveillance centers. FXB HIV/AIDS projects in India have expanded enormously in the past 13 years since we first established FXB Homes for children affected by AIDS in Goa in 1991. Today, FXB India-the only Non-Governmental Organization (NGO) in the field of HIV/AIDS and Human Rights present in all 35 States and Union Territories of India-aims to fight the AIDS pandemic there, and thus prevent the millions of orphans that the disease caused in Southern Africa. The prevention, education, treatment programs implemented by us till date has been able to benefit more than 235,000 people directly and another 860,000 indirectly.

## OUR PROGRAMS ARE BROAD AND EXTENSIVE

1. Orphans and Vulnerable Children Projects include caring for the children of sex workers, protecting street children and training and care for orphans Projects for school children and non formal education and awareness for children not attending schools tend to minimize the high risk behavior amongst them.
2. Targeted Interventions with 'At Risk' marginalized Groups. Included as risk groups are migrant workers away from home for long periods of time, fishermen who do the same, slum dwellers, and injection drug users. Since FXB is in all the states of India, we are able to sensitize and target both the migrants and their families back home in a cost-effective manner.
3. Prevention of Mother-to-Child Transmission of HIV/AIDS with an extensive outreach program with a referral

network to ensure the maximum coverage and ante-natal care referral along with the quality HIV counseling and testing for pregnant women

4. Awareness and Preventive Education Outreach are innovative HIV/AIDS education and mass awareness programs, for example, for barbers and their clientele, interventions in pubs, bars and wine shops and HIV/AIDS counseling by telephone.
5. FXB Voluntary Counseling Center and sexually transmitted diseases (STD) Clinic: These centers provide the quality counseling and testing/referral for screening of STDs and treatment for the most important core high risk and bridging groups of the target population.
6. Workplace Interventions. HIV/AIDS education programs are brought into the workplaces such as technology parks and jute mills and other industries.
7. HIV/AIDS Care and Treatment: FXB Centers for HIV/AIDS Care and Treatment have well trained Medical personnel coupled with the health facilities to deliver effective care to the target population in most cost effective manner without compromising on the quality of care.

Some of the above activities are well established in some states; in others they are just beginning. The projects featured on the web site give a sampling of the all the projects. HIV/AIDS in India-social challenges faced by HIV +ve couples.

**Background:** The ignorance of society and health care providers, lack of social support organisations and lethargy of the legal system causes many HIV +ve couples to face social and cultural problems which cannot be discussed and remain simmering below the surface. Method: During periodical counseling sessions at the AIDS clinic, in metropolis of South Bombay 200 couples were recruited in which at least one partner was HIV +ve. The attempt was made to study and categorise the challenges faced by them and classify them.

***Result***: The frequency of sexual relation decreased drastically. Most couples face guilt and denial and the practice of safer sex was denied by majority of couples. Condom was blamed for decreasing pleasure, causing irritation, not being 100% protective and was looked upon with suspicions. The fright, guilt and the prospect of living with HIV cannot often be discussed with the spouse as the family infringes on their privacy with their personal opinions, taboos, & alternative therapies. Since most of couples were newly married (80%) the prospect of remaining infertile or not seeing their children grow into adulthood was frightening. Negative elder children were taken up by the immediate family, but +ve children and their health responsibility remained with their sick parents. Since it would expose them to gossip & speculation, adoption was not considered a viable option by most couples. Decreasing economic productivity and increasing health care cost remained a major hurdle.

Health benefits and insurance were flatly denied. Alternative employment was difficult to obtain and many seropositive people found themselves out of employment without notifications & salary. Many orphanages now take up and place negative children, for adoption whose parents have died of HIV/AIDS, but positive children were victim of social stigmatisations. Female spouses suffered most since they were comparatively less educated, dependent on the family & faced sexual harassment at the work place & within their joint family settings too. Conclusions: In India which is estimated to have highest number of HIV +ve individuals in the world; effective counseling services, social support organisations, voluntary legal services, organised orphanages & motivated joint family systems will reduce considerably the impact of HIV +ve couples on HIV/AIDS epidemic.

Smile Foundation and Child Survival India [CSI] has come together for a project on named Nanhe Sapne (Little Dreams) in the most vulnerable areas of Delhi, the capital of India. The project takes the responsibility of providing care, support and mainstreaming of HIV inflicted, affected and vulnerable children. The focus, undoubtedly, is on children inflicted with HIV, children of HIV inflicted parents as well as vulnerable children living on streets, including child labours.

Resource Centre for Sexual Health and HIV/AIDS [RCSHA], New Delhi came forward as the technical partner for the project.

## About the Partner

Child Survival India (CSI) is an organization established in the year 1991 by a group of young professionals with an aim to help the marginalized and vulnerable sections of community to find new avenues and alternatives.

The organization is primarily working in the field of Health (RCH, HIV/AIDS prevention, support for HIV/AIDS infected & affected); gender sensitization for rural (school) student's teachers and their parents; adolescent girls and boys; literacy, legal issues and organizing mahila panchayat for empowerment of rural women.

## The Project

Nanhe Sapne (Little Dreams) is the project name initiated by Smile Foundation and CSI. It will take up the responsibility of providing care, support and mainstreaming of HIV inflicted, affected and vulnerable children. The focus, undoubtedly, is on children inflicted with HIV, children of HIV inflicted parents as well as vulnerable children living on streets, including child labours.

The target areas for the project Nanhe Sapne (Little Dreams) are few of the most needy and deserving localities of Delhi, such as Narela, Holambi Khurd, Holambi Kalan, Kherakhud, Bhorgarh, Sanjay Gandhi Transport Nagar and Rohini.

A brief description of a few of the target project areas are as follows:

Kherakhud is a rural village located in outskirts of Delhi, about 20 kms from Main G. T Karnal Road. CSI is operating its regional office from this place which is also functioning as the joint project office.

Sanjay Gandhi Transport Nagar is in North West Delhi near the GT Karnal Road Bypass. It is a major halt point for truck drivers, helpers and cleaners. It is surrounded by a number of slums like Seemapuri and Jahangirpuri. The area is also dominated by transport company owners, brokers, loaders, labourers, petrol pump staff, mechanics, road side eateries and tea stall owners as well as female sex workers. All these made this locality vulnerable and hence most deserving for attention.

Holambi Kalan is situated in North West part of Delhi near Holambi Village. It is divided into two geographical phases-Phase I and II with 7200 houses in each, i.e. 43,000 individuals in one phase approximately. The people here have been relocated around 3 years back from in and around Delhi. The majority of the communities are migrants from states like Bihar, Bengal and Uttar Pradesh, working as daily wager earners with an average salary of Rs 3000 to 4000 per month.

Narela Industrial Area is surrounded by Narela Village. CSI already has a good presence here. Smile Foundation and CSI have done a couple of community based short term activities in recent past.

The project aims will identify and cover all vulnerable/at-risk and infected children, enabling them to lead a healthy and productive life. The objective of the project is to:

- Help HIV/AIDS affected children to cope with HIV infection in family and also their own infections.
- Increase knowledge on HIV/AIDS issues and reduce risk behaviors like unsafe sex and drug abuse practices amongst the vulnerable children.
- To prepare the families and communities to take care of HIV/AIDS affected children.
- To provide Non-formal education to vulnerable children and mainstream these children to some formal government school, as best as possible.
- To facilitate Vocational Training, at some suitable training institution(s) run by Govt./NGOs, to such children after they have completed NFE (non-formal education); their regular follow-up and facilitating their engagement in some gainful activities/employment with help from Training Institutions.

Target beneficiaries of the Project:

- 50 HIV/AIDS affected children,
- 360 vulnerable children (5-16 years) in targeted community's *e.g* child laborers, street children, out of school children and adolescent.

- 50 girls being covered only in PPTCT( Prevention from parents to child transmission) workshops (6 proposed)

HIV infected/affected children shall be provided with the following:

- Antiretroviral treatment through linkages with govt. run programme
- Pediatric disclosure: talking to children about HIV/AIDS
- Supportive care (counseling, emotional support, providing education, health, nutritional therapy, gainful engagements etc.)
- HIV prevention education
- Facilitate admission to Vocational Training Centers; mainstreaming out-of-school children to some formal schools-after remedial education support; provide uniform, books and reading materials.
- To provide school fees, toiletries and nutrition supports besides certain other provisions like rentals and electricity bills etc.
- To provide funeral expenses in case of a death
- Arrange outings, festival celebrations, creativity workshops, special workshops on child sexual abuse, HIV/AIDS transmission.
- Life skills training (in self defense, negotiation skills etc.) for affected children.

For vulnerable children (street and working children, adolescent girls, youths (14-19 years):

- Establish learning centers for street/working children
- Conduct life skills sessions on peer pressures, conflict resolution, sexual abuse, HIV/AIDS etc for working/ street children (adolescents)
- Organize monthly health check up camps and provide follow up & health services
- Special workshops on early age marriage, condom negotiations and prevention of parent to child transmission of HIV for adolescent girls

- Special long term programmes for adolescent girls imparting life skills integrated with vocational skill training
- Special workshops on STIs, HIV/AIDS and condom usage for youths.

**Special Focus**

- 50 girls being covered only in PPTCT (Prevention from Parents to Child Transmission) Programme under the project
- Special long term programmes for adolescent girls imparting life skills integrated with vocational skill training
- Special design to make the programme self sustainable in the communities and localities.

At the age of four, Gopi has seen first his father and then his mother succumb to HIV/AIDS. Gopi and his sister Siri have not been tested yet but are most likely to be infected. They live with their grandmother in Vijayawada.

On the surface, Vijayawada appears to be the quintessential bustling Indian city—a booming centre of commerce and industry. But behind this seeming prosperity lurks a disturbing threat. The National AIDS Control Organisation (NACO) has identified this part of Andhra Pradesh as one of the highest-risk zones for the prevalence of HIV/AIDS, where the epidemic is rapidly crossing over to the general population from high-risk groups.

More alarming are estimates that suggest that the city has over 30,000 AIDS orphans. Parentless and homeless, civil society organisations working in Vijayawada say many of these children have been forced to drop out of school and beg on the streets.

India today is home to the largest number of AIDS orphans in the world (the UN estimates children orphaned by AIDS as those under the age of 18 who have lost one or both parents to the disease). While India's AIDS orphan crisis is not as dire as Africa's, it is on the trajectory Africa was during the last decade. With widespread migrant labour, prostitution and a stigma about sexually-transmitted diseases causing an explosion in AIDS cases, India is expected to become the next epicentre of the AIDS orphan crisis. Though there are no government figures in the country for the number of children affected by AIDS, World Bank estimates suggest that the number of children in India orphaned by AIDS is approaching 2 million.

While the statistics on HIV infections in India is the subject of ongoing controversy, what is undeniable is that India is at a critical juncture of the HIV/AIDS pandemic. Despite the low sero-prevalence rate, in absolute terms India is second only to South Africa in the number of people living with HIV/AIDS. This is compounded by the fact that there are several localised sub-epidemics in states such as Maharashtra, Andhra Pradesh, Tamil Nadu, Manipur, Karnataka and Nagaland.

The escalating AIDS crisis is leaving an unprecedented number of children orphaned with little or no adult protection and care. The proportion of orphaned children is expected to double in the next five years and remain exceptionally high until 2020 or 2030. Given the long incubation period between infection and the onset of symptoms, the epidemic's impact will linger for decades even if the rate of new infections is brought under control. The orphan crisis is also likely to have an impact on the country's economic and social fabric.

The odds against AIDS-orphaned children are staggering. These children are vulnerable to a number of risks ranging from social exclusion and economic deprivation to illiteracy, malnutrition and exploitation. They are also at increased risk of contracting sexually-transmitted diseases, abuse and drug use, with many young girls turning to prostitution in order to survive. AIDS orphans are often shunned by their communities; many are denied property rights and rights to inheritance. Those who cannot be taken in by their relatives end up living on the streets.

Children in HIV/AIDS-affected households begin to suffer even before a parent or caregiver has died. Household income plummets. Schooling is often interrupted and many children are forced to drop out either to care for a sick parent or to earn money. Depression and alienation are common. Another worrying phenomenon is the emergence of child-headed households. With parents gone, children have to take on the responsibility of earning money, looking after younger siblings and running households. The threats and challenges these children face is compounded by the emotional trauma of losing parents and the stigma associated with the disease, which marks them out as a new class of untouchables.

Experts say that India's crisis is becoming acute in part because the country has no national policy to specifically address the impact of HIV/AIDS on children. The plight of AIDS orphans goes virtually unnoticed as most of them are being left to fend for themselves. Intervention options for providing care and support to orphans in the country are limited. India has little experience with community-based care, and institutional care is often relied upon as the most common form of intervention. However, even the number of orphanages providing short-term care for AIDS orphans is insufficient. In Andhra Pradesh, for example, a state with a population of 79 million, there is only one orphanage with a capacity for 20 children.

A more fundamental concern is whether there is sufficient commitment at the government level to combating the epidemic. As the epidemic spreads, the battle against AIDS is mired by a lack of consensus on the extent of the pandemic, the right strategy to combat it, and how to deal frankly with the issue of sexuality. The Indian government has been criticised for clinging to the idea that the epidemic is limited to 'high-risk groups' like sex workers, drug users and truck drivers. But this approach no longer reflects the reality of at least some Indian states, where the epidemic is in the general population.

With regard to anti-retroviral (ARV) drugs, despite the fact that India is a major producer of cheap generic copies of many HIV/AIDS drugs that are being sold all over the world, ARVs are affordable and accessible only to a tiny fraction of people in need of treatment. India's spending on public health has also, historically, been very low. India spends almost a ninth of what Uganda spends per person on HIV treatment and prevention. On a more positive note though, earlier this year NACO announced that it would more than double its annual budget to Rs 4.2 billion (US$ 96 million) to combat the disease.

Supporting and protecting children affected by HIV/AIDS requires generating a sense of shared responsibility and vision.

The debilitating impact of children affected by AIDS needs to be countered by strong and nurturing community and family support. Orphanages are the least effective form of care for reducing AIDS-related vulnerability among children.

Interventions must respond to the need for large-scale and long-term effects that both directly and indirectly impact on orphaned children. Recent guidelines developed by UNICEF focus on child-centred, family and community-oriented, and human rights-based principles. This calls for building national systems of care that support local coping, establish and enhance community systems of care, and strengthen partnerships between various government and non-government organisations.

Fundamental steps in building a supportive environment include involving children and families affected by HIV/AIDS in care and treatment strategies; increasing awareness of the impact of HIV/AIDS on children and families; and reducing fear, ignorance, denial and discrimination by increasing access to information, challenging myths and transforming the public perception about HIV/AIDS.

In a country with over 1 billion people, 2 million might seem like a small figure. But playing the numbers game is counterproductive—and perhaps callous. We need to move beyond feeling beleaguered to feeling outraged by the unacceptable suffering of these children. Because behind the numbers are young people whose lives are at stake—a generation that's being denied its hopes, aspirations and rights.

## HIV/AIDS

"We believe that children have the right to information and services to help them avoid HIV.

### Objectives for the India Programme

- To reduce the vulnerability of children and young people to HIV infection in project intervention areas through informed choices.
- To influence policy makers on successful approaches to reduce children's vulnerability.

- To ameliorate the impact of HIV/AIDS on children affected by or living with HIV/AIDS in high prevalence areas through increased awareness and support from families, communities and state, through addressing discrimination, poverty, property rights and access to health and education services.

**Programmes**

The scale of the HIV/AIDS epidemic in India is becoming recognised. In five states (Maharashtra, Karnataka, Andhra Pradesh, Tamil Nadu and Manipur) HIV/AIDS prevalence is already greater than 1% in Ante Natal Clinics, the measure used to indicate that the infection has crossed to the general population. The issue is high on the donor agenda and the government has established the National AIDS Control Organisation (NACO), which promotes health awareness work and campaigns and also has state cells.

Despite this, our research on vulnerability and impact of HIV/AIDS on children in India shows that access to information alone does not change behaviour patterns of children, particularly those who are most vulnerable (such as children living in the streets, children who work, children involved in sex work, girls forced into sexual relations for religious reasons). There is little peer-led awareness work. As well, many interventions focus only on school-going children. Another issue is that often programmes do not challenge either the unfriendly, judgemental attitudes of health workers or the perception that HIV/AIDS is essentially a health issue and not linked to social factors. It is important to support children develop their own messages to their peers on HIV/AIDS prevention and impact, messages there are culturally and age-sensitive. As the epidemic spreads so will the number of children affected by HIV/AIDS increase. This will be manifest in issues of discrimination, children being unable to continue in school because of the costs of treating dying parents, being forced into work or looking after younger siblings. Challenging discrimination can be developed through mainstreaming HIV/AIDS work through all of our projects, building the understanding, sensitivity and capacity of partners work effectively with communities.

## Some Highlights of Our Work

As of now, within Save the Children, two of the zonal programmes are addressing the issue of HIV/AIDS. In North West India, this issue is important as both Leh and Kargil are potentially vulnerable to HIV infection on account of a huge army presence, high degree of migration and truckers movement. Given this scenario, the North West India Programme has decided to create awareness among different stakeholders as its main area of intervention on the issue.

Along with the Leh Nutritional Project we have developed a new approach to awareness raising and sensitization in relation to reproductive health and sexually transmitted diseases. Peer education and support is one of the key components of our efforts at creating awareness and behavioural changes among the community members. The project has developed a training manual on adolescent reproductive sexual health, which has been used widely by the team during field testing and has been found very effective. In addition, training workshops have been conducted on adolescent reproductive sexual health for children leading to increased awareness about health issues and HIV/AIDS.

The state of Andhra Pradesh, in South India has one of the highest prevalence rates of HIV/AIDS. We have documented several case studies of women and children who are infected and affected by HIV/AIDS to understand their needs and thereby inform our future interventions.

These case studies would also be used towards influencing the policy developed by the state government. Our work with children in the context of HIV/AIDS informs us of the urgent need for developing IEC materials that are child friendly. We are currently moving towards addressing this issue as a cross-cutting theme in all our ongoing programmes in Andhra Pradesh and Orissa. For those who are affected or infected by HIV/AIDS, interventions are meaningful and effective, only if they are holistic and help them to cope with the disease in such a manner that they are able to lead their every day lives without any discrimination. We therefore feel the need to work towards ensuring that children who are infected or affected are not excluded from education and other services.

Save the Children has used innovative methods for reaching out to the community members to discuss sensitive issues such as HIV/AIDS. Theater for Development is one such tool. Its significance lies in the fact that using drama as a medium of expression, children are able to reach adults and create awareness among the community on this issue. Other activities include individual counseling for school teachers, setting up of medical camps and awareness raising of safe sexual health practices through distribution of Communication material on behavioral change.

For the India Country Programme, the issue of HIV/AIDS is fairly new. However, our current work especially with children who are infected or affected by HIV/AIDS has given us insights into the needs of the children. Our efforts to address the issue as a cross cutting one are significant as they have huge potential to influence not only the work of Save the Children in rest of the country but also of other organisations including the government. This will be a main focus of work for us in the future.

In 2002, ILO (India) initiated a study to understand the socio-economic impact of HIV/AIDS on infected persons and their families, particularly on women and children. The findings of this report which was published recently are significant because of the sensitivity with which the study was carried out. Conducted in collaboration with the network of people living with HIV/AIDS (PLWHA), the study underlines the adverse economic impact of HIV/AIDS, and the trauma arising from stigma, discrimination and ostracism.

The study focussed on four Indian states-Delhi, Maharashtra, Manipur and Tamilnadu-chosen because of the high-prevalence of the disease. The data was collected by the networks of people living with HIV/AIDS in Delhi (DNP+), Manipur MNP+), Maharashtra (NMP+) and the Positive Women's Network of South India (PWN). All these organisations maintained the confidentiality of PLWHA.

The most disturbing aspect of the study's findings pertains to the impact of HIV/AIDS on women. Conducted amongst 292 people, of whom 42 per cent were women, the study reveals that 74 per cent of the HIV positive women faced a lot of discrimination, hardships and responsibilities. Ironically, it was the family of the infected person that discriminated the most compared to other sections of society. Women felt betrayed by this lack of understanding from the family despite the fact that they were (and are) the prime care-givers, doing all the household chores uncomplainingly.

The women were also deeply hurt by the aspersions cast on the their sexual lives by their in-laws, despite the awareness that Indian women in general have no control over their sexual expression. Although a majority of women were infected through their husbands, they were blamed for their death. In many cases, the woman was accused of causing her husband's illness, and either disowned or deserted by her in-laws.

The children of infected parents are also heavily discriminated against-they are verbally abused and taunted and not allowed to play with other children. Although there was no evidence of forced child labour, as much as 35 per cent of the children were denied basic amenities and about 17 per cent were forced to take on petty jobs to augment the family income.

Education is considered an important tool for attitudinal change. In keeping with this view, the study found that a relatively high level of education among the infected (and by implication their families) had an impact on the extent of discrimination they experienced. Fifty-nine per cent of postgraduate respondents faced discrimination compared to 74 per cent of those educated up to school level and 71.42 per cent of those who were illiterate. Women were more vulnerable, with 17.21 per cent being illiterate compared to 11.18 per cent of the men. While 22 per cent of the men were graduates and above, only eight per cent of the women were graduates and above.

The study also indicates that the average monthly income of a PLWHA was about Rs 1,117, whereas average monthly expenditure was Rs 3,185. In many cases, this gap was met by loans or sale of assets leading to an increase of indebtedness averaging Rs.4,818 per family. While medical costs varied in accordance with the stage of the illness, the fact that HIV infected persons have to go for regular check-ups underscored the economic impact of the infection. The ILO study has also shown and reinforced the fact that HIV infection cuts across all barriers of class and religion. Besides, the findings also reveal that a majority of the infected people is from the highly productive and reproductive age group. There can be no doubt that well designed interventions are urgently required to reduce the socio-economic costs for PLWHA. And equally important is the realisation that discrimination against PLWHA is a denial of their basic fundamental rights. Unless policymakers facilitate a supportive environment that encourages HIV positive people to reveal their status and seek help, India may soon have a still larger number of people affected by HIV/AIDS.

**Comments by Global Strategies for HIV Prevention:** Most of you probably heard or saw a recent new report on issues related to the safety and effectiveness of nevirapine to prevent HIV transmission from mothers to children (PMTCT). It is important to understand whether the recent news report impacts on current recommendations for the use of nevirapine for PMTCT in developing countries.

Some facts:

1. This is not new news. Questions were asked by the scientific community following the publication in 1999 of the initial study known as HIVNET 012, a clinical study performed in pregnant women and their infants in Uganda. The scientific community knew that the study was not designed as a clinical study directed towards FDA approval of nevirapine. This would have required a greater stringency in quality control, monitoring and data collection.

   Thus most of us concluded that additional studies would be required to confirm the effectiveness and safety of nevirapine. Nevertheless, the result of the study, a 50% reduction in HIV transmission to infants, was considered to be of such great significance that recommendations could be made for the use of nevirapine for PMTCT while additional studies were being pursued. Historically, this was in keeping with making life saving drugs available while still under evaluation-some thing that all advocates and activists for AIDS argued strongly for.

2. Current recommendations for the use of nevirapine for PMTCT are not based on the HIVNET 012 study alone. In fact, there are now 17 clinical trials throughout the world, conducted by multiple investigators, from many different countries, using either single dose nevirapine or combination of other antiretroviral drugs along with single-dose nevirapine, to evaluate safety and effectiveness in PMTCT.
3. Seven on the 17 clinical trials now show that single dose nevirapine for mothers and infants or single-dose in combination with other antiretroviral drugs, reduces HIV transmission, in some instances by as over 90%.
4. None of the 17 clinical trials raise any major safety concern regarding the use of single dose nevirapine for PMTCT. No fatalities have been attributed to single dose nevirapine in any of these studies. Nevirapine can cause significant rash, liver disease and occasional fatalities when used as chronic therapy to treat HIV infection in either men or nonpregnant women. This is not how nevirapine is used for PMTCT. Health care workers have been aware of these complications for over 5 years.
5. Based on safety and effectiveness, single dose nevirapine or single-dose nevirapine in combination with other antiretroviral drugs, its use is recommended by all international health agencies and national governments conducting PMTCT programs. This includes the World Health Organization, UNAIDS, the US Public Health Service including the CDC, British and European national health organizations, the International AIDS Society, the Elizabeth Glaser Pediatric AIDS Foundation and Global Strategies for HIV Prevention. In addition, all countries conducting PMTCT programs include the addition of single-dose nevirapine as an appropriate approach to PMTCT in resource poor countries.

The issue of resistance to nevirapine and its impact on subsequent use in HIV-infected women has also been debated. Several important facts need to be considered.

1. Nevirapine resistance occurs even with single-dose nevirapine given to mothers. This resistance is transient and there is no evidence that it prevents the effectiveness of nevirapine in subsequent pregnancies. Health care workers have known about nevirapine resistance for over five years and have taken this into consideration in making recommendations for PMTCT.
2. All drugs used to treat HIV infection result in resistance. HIV rapidly mutates and resistance is inevitable. The use of combination antiretroviral drugs, which controls viral replication, reduces but does not eliminate the possibility of resistance. It is not logical to withhold nevirapine to save the life of an infant based on theoretical concerns regarding subsequent responses to therapy. Resistance can develop whether nevirapine is used for PMTCT or for treatment of HIV infection.
3. WHO, UNAIDS and other international and national health organizations recommend combination drug therapy to treat HIV-infected adults who meet certain criteria for initiation of treatment. Several low-cost regimens include nevirapine as recommended therapy in resource poor countries. Resistance to nevirapine can occur with any of the recommended regimens for treatment of HIV-infected individuals.
4. The "threat of resistance" arguments are backwards. The greatest threat for the development of widespread nevirapine resistance is not from its use as single-dose nevirapine for PMTCT in several hundreds of thousands of pregnant women. Rather widespread nevirapine resistance is more likely to result from its use with combination drugs to treat millions of HIV-infected individuals worldwide and could jeopardize its use for PMTCT.
5. Withholding nevirapine, on the theoretical basis of blunting a subsequent response if used in combination therapy to treat HIV infection, would result in HIV infection and subsequent death of hundreds of thousands of infants for whom no other options are available. In contrast, over 17 antiretroviral drugs are available which

can be used in various combinations to treat HIV infection if resistance occurs. In most resource poor countries the only option for preventing HIV-infected babies is single-dose nevirapine.

**Conclusion**

So what is behind the recent publication of information that has been known for over 4 years by the FDA, the international AIDS community, WHO, UNAIDS and the scientific community? Basically the media report deceptively presents itself as new information.

Importantly however, the clinical research and scientific community have gone far beyond the 1999 HIVNET 012 report and have conducted multiple additional studies to confirm both the effectiveness and safety of nevirapine used either as a single dose for PMTCT or in combination with other antiretroviral drugs. Many of these studies are completed and confirm the safety and effectiveness of single-dose nevirapine and its much greater effectiveness when used with other antiretroviral agents to reduce HIV transmission by over 90%. The media report fails to acknowledge these advances.

It is absolutely essential that PMTCT programs move forward quickly to save the lives of infants from fatal HIV infection. Once an opportunity is missed to prevent HIV infection, one cannot go back and eradicate an already established and ultimately fatal infection.

We all want to treat with the best combination antiretroviral drugs available to prevent as many infections of babies as possible. We also want to optimally treat the mother's HIV infection. But as we move toward that goal, single dose nevirapine may be the only option for resource poor countries until more effective therapy becomes available.

Global Strategies for HIV Prevention will continue to support programs in resource poor countries using single-dose nevirapine alone or in combination with other antiretroviral therapy to reduce the number of newly HIV-infected infants, which number 1,800 each day. In 1997, a clinical trial known as HIVNET 012 was begun in Uganda to address the developing world's urgent need for safe, effective and affordable regimens to prevent mother-to-infant transmission of HIV. The study was funded by the National Institute of Allergy and Infectious Diseases (NIAID) of the National Institutes of Health (NIH) and conducted by co-investigators from The Johns Hopkins University and Makerere University in Kampala, Uganda.

The purpose of HIVNET 012 was to examine whether a simple, inexpensive regimen of the drug nevirapine could effectively block mother-to-infant HIV transmission. In the study, both mother and baby were treated with a single dose of nevirapine, a drug licensed for the treatment of HIV-infected adults and children in the United States.

The researchers found that this intervention reduced the risk of mother-to-infant HIV transmission by approximately 50 percent. The results of this landmark study were published in The Lancet in 1999.

The HIVNET 012 nevirapine regimen subsequently has been endorsed by the World Health Organization (WHO), the Joint United Nations Programme on AIDS (UNAIDS) and other international organizations. NIAID stands by the accuracy of the results of HIVNET 012.

The simple and cost-effective nevirapine regimen has been used in developing countries to prevent HIV infection in thousands of infants; it represents a major public health advance and is one of the true success stories in HIV prevention.

The results of HIVNET 012, including the safety and effectiveness of the nevirapine regimen, have been subjected to multiple reviews. In every instance, the initial conclusions of the HIVNET 012 investigators have been found to be correct. In addition, findings of other studies conducted in the United States and internationally have consistently supported the results of HIVNET 012.

Because of the striking results of HIVNET 012, in 2001 the manufacturer of nevirapine decided to apply to the U.S. Food and Drug Administration (FDA) for an expanded indication for nevirapine in the United States to include use of the drug to prevent mother-to-infant transmission of HIV. As part of the evaluation of the HIVNET 012 trial for this new indication, the conclusions of HIVNET 012 were re-affirmed as valid. Certain aspects of the collection of some of the primary data, however, did not strictly conform to FDA regulatory requirements. For this reason, the study could not serve as a single pivotal trial leading to an expanded indication.

As noted above, NIAID and NIH initiated several reviews and re-reviews of HIVNET 012. These reviews identified procedural flaws in the study that led NIAID to implement improvements in the conduct of clinical research it supports both in the United States and abroad. We understand that certain previously recognized criticisms of the conduct of HIVNET 012 have re-emerged, but stress strongly that throughout multiple reviews, the overall conclusions regarding the safety and efficacy of single-dose nevirapine in this setting have remained intact.

Moreover, NIH has contracted the Institute of Medicine (IOM), part of the National Academy of Sciences, to conduct an additional independent review of HIVNET 012. The results of the IOM review are anticipated in March 2005. NIAID is confident that the previous conclusions regarding the integrity of the HIVNET 012 data will be upheld.

The reduction of perinatal HIV transmission by the use of the readily accessible, inexpensive nevirapine regimen studied by the HIVNET 012 investigators represents a major public health advance for developing countries. No new data exist to suggest that current recommendations regarding use of this regimen should be changed, and we urge clinicians and policymakers to continue to heed the current WHO and UNAIDS guidance on single-dose nevirapine.

Media inquiries can be directed to the NIAID OCPL media group at 301-402-1663.

NIAID is a component of the National Institutes of Health, an agency of the U.S. Department of Health and Human Services. NIAID supports basic and applied research to prevent, diagnose and treat infectious diseases such as HIV/AIDS and other sexually transmitted infections, influenza, tuberculosis, malaria and illness from potential agents of bioterrorism. NIAID also supports research on transplantation and immune-related illnesses, including autoimmune disorders, asthma and allergies. Articles from the Associated Press (AP) and other media sources appear to raise serious questions about the use of single-dose nevirapine to prevent mother-to-child transmission of HIV in resource poor countries. Although there is no new information about the safety and effectiveness of the use of this prevention strategy, the articles appear to raise questions about how the results of a study in Uganda were reported by the National Institute of Allergy and Infectious Diseases.

Project Inform, a national HIV/AIDS treatment information and advocacy organization that has served hundreds of thousands of people living with HIV since its inception in 1985, contends it would be an enormous disservice to people struggling to fight HIV worldwide to conclude from these stories that this use of nevirapine should be stopped or curtailed.

There are currently only two scientifically proven regimens for the treatment of mother-to-child transmission. The first, and oldest, requires that the mother be treated with AZT for six weeks prior to delivery and given intravenous AZT during delivery, followed by six weeks of AZT given to the infant. The second approach is a single dose of the drug nevirapine given once to the mother and once to the infant. Both regimens have demonstrated approximately equal effectiveness in reducing the risk of transmitting HIV to the infant. It is self evident that the second approach offers many practical advantages over the first, including a major cost advantage. In many resource poor settings, the regimen based solely on AZT is not even feasible, given the common lack of health care infrastructure and limited funds for treatment. Also, as a general rule, a single dose of nevirapine creates fewer side effects for both mother and infant. These factors have made the use of single-dose nevirapine

The study in Uganda mentioned in the AP article and related stories did not reach any conclusions that should discourage the use of single-dose nevirapine. This approach has been used in tens of thousands of pregnant women in studies and in common usage. The scientific data shows it to be both safe and effective and far more convenient than alternative regimens in resource poor settings. There are potentially significant toxicities associated with long-term use of nevirapine, as there are with many drugs used in the treatment of AIDS, but these long-term effects are rarely seen in single-dose, short-term use.

The Ugandan study and other studies have demonstrated that a single dose of nevirapine can sometimes produce resistance to the drug. It is incorrect to say that this precludes effective treatment for HIV for the mother or infant in the future. Unfortunately, the AP story gives the reader this mistaken impression.

There have been three major studies of single dose nevirapine in recent years: (1) the HIVNET 012 study in Uganda; (2) PACTG 316 in the US, Europe, Brazil and the Bahamas; and (3) the SAINT trial in South Africa. Collectively, these studies involved more than 1600 HIV-infected women and their infants. No significant laboratory or clinical toxicity was found in any of these studies, again contrary to the impression given in recent press articles. There is, therefore, no scientific reason to delay or halt the use of this regimen.

The Ugandan Study, HIVNET 012, was initiated in 1999 as a "proof of concept study." It was also meant to be a pilot exercise for Ugandan researchers. It was not a study designed to meet US FDA standards. However, when the study was stopped early because of its high success rate in preventing transmission to the infants, the manufacturer of nevirapine, Boehringer Ingelheim, unexpectedly sought to use the data to seek a new label indication for the drug in the US.

This had the effect of retroactively imposing the FDA standards and requirements for a formal proof of efficacy study on HIVNET 012. It was a standard the study was never designed to meet and subsequent reviews of the data found many errors in data collection.

The AP press report presented a highly exaggerated view of these errors, suggesting that the study may have had "thousands" of serious adverse events. In fact, the final review of the study showed no such thing. There were 37 adverse events experienced by women or infant.

The world currently faces the greatest pandemic in its history. The UN reports that as many as 1900 children are infected with HIV daily. No vaccine appears likely any time soon. Treatment is difficult, expensive and often out of reach. Every available tool must be used to try to reduce the rate of new infections. The use of single-dose nevirapine, like currently available alternatives, may not be a perfect solution to blocking mother-to-child transmission of HIV, but it is a useful and effective tool in its current form.

Additional research is underway testing other, newer methods, including combinations of nevirapine and AZT, combinations of other drugs, and single pill interventions using other drugs. We may speculate that one or another of these alternative approaches might be superior to single-dose nevirapine or pose fewer risks, but we cannot reach such a conclusion until the appropriate clinical trials are completed. For now, single-dose nevirapine remains a critically important tool.

The questions raised about the Uganda trial do not ultimately raise real concerns about the safety or effectiveness of single-dose nevirapine. Exaggerated reports and emotional language in the media can only exacerbate the difficult challenges facing the world in its efforts to bring HIV infection under control in resource poor settings.

To the extent that media stories about the Ugandan single-dose nevirapine study cause pregnant women or their governments to doubt the value of this approach to prevention, they are only adding to the problem. Whether it is possible, appropriate, or necessary for studies conducted in such settings to fully replicate the standards expected of research in the US or Europe is an important question which must be addressed as more studies are conducted in such international settings. But it is not a question that should be used to delay or thwart access to proven solutions.

## GLOBAL AIDS

The United Nations' Children's Fund (UNICEF) late Thursday (Nov 19) hailed a study done in Zambia on a cheap, common antibiotic that greatly reduces the death rate among children with the AIDS virus as "a major breakthrough."

The research findings of Britain's Department for International Development (DFID) "represent a major breakthrough, and has the potential to save the lives of hundreds of thousands of children each year," UNICEF said in a statement.

In the research, to be published in next Saturday's issue of The Lancet, Co-trimoxazole, a combination of two drugs that is one of the cheapest antibiotics in the world, was used in a test that involved 534

Zambian children aged under 15 who had the Human Immunodeficiency Virus (HIV).

Half of the children were given the drug each day in the form of an oral dose; the other half were given a harmless look alike called a placebo. When researchers did a follow up 19 months later, they found that 74 (28 percent) of the children in the co-trimoxazole group had died, while 112 (42 percent) had died in the placebo group.

The findings were so remarkable that the study was discontinued on ethical grounds. The placebo group was immediately put on co-trimoxazole.

The clinical reason for the success is unclear, but it is thought the drug combats pneumonia and tuberculosis bacteria that commonly claims the lives of people whose immune systems have been wrecked by HIV.

'UNICEF has been hopeful that co-trimoxazole could work to prolong children's lives, and now that we have the hard evidence, the challenge is to reach as many children as we can, and immediately," UNICEF said in its statement.

"This cheap, widely available drug makes it possible to ensure that every child who needs it, can get it," it said.

On November 24, following the above report, the following joint statement was issued by WHO, UNAIDS and UNICEF.

WHO, UNAIDS and UNICEF modify recommendations for cotrimoxazole prophylaxis in children.

Joint WHO/UNAIDS/UNICEF statement on use of cotrimoxazole as prophylaxis in HIV exposed and HIV infected children

## Statement on use of Cotrimoxazole Prophylaxis

**22 November 2004:** WHO, UNAIDS and UNICEF, guided by recent evidence, have agreed to modify as an interim the current recommendations (1) for cotrimoxazole prophylaxis in children. This is based upon recent trial data from Zambia (2).

These data and other new evidence will be reviewed in early 2005 by an expert committee convened to revise and update the recommendations for cotrimoxazole for adults and children. Cotrimoxazole remains important even with increasing access to ART, as it use can improve survival independently of specific HIV treatment.

Current recommendations suggest it should be used before children require ARVs because it may even postpone the time at which ART needs to be started.

Prophylactic dosing with cotrimoxazole for HIV infected children with any sign or symptoms suggestive of HIV is a key intervention that should be offered as part of a basic package of care to reduce morbidity and mortality.

Cotrimoxazole prophylaxis is also a crucial potentially life saving intervention that should be given to all HIV exposed children born to HIV-infected mothers, in settings where HIV infection status cannot be reliably confirmed in the first 18 months of life.

Cotrimoxazole is a widely available antibiotic that is available in syrup and solid formulations at low-cost in most settings, including resource limited settings. It is highly effective for the treatment and prevention of Pneumocystis pneumonia. In HIV infected children it also offers protection against other infections, this remains important even with increasing access to ARV treatment.

Greater advocacy for the use of cotrimoxazole prophylaxis in children is urgently required.

Who should get cotrimoxazole:

- All HIV exposed children (children born to HIV infected mothers) from 4-6 weeks of age (whether or not part of a prevention of mother-to-child transmission [PMTCT] programme)

- Any child identified as HIV-infected with any clinical signs or symptoms suggestive of HIV, regardless of age or CD4 count.

**How Long should Cotrimoxazole be Given:** Cotrimoxazole is required to be taken as follows:

- HIV exposed children-until HIV infection has been definitively ruled out AND the mother is no longer breastfeeding
- HIV infected children-indefinitely where ARV treatment is not yet available.
- Where ARV treatment is being given-cotrimoxazole can be stopped only once clinical or immunological indicators confirm restoration of the immune system for 6 months or more. With current evidence it is not yet clear if cotrimoxazole continues to provide protection after immune restoration is achieved.

Under what circumstances should cotrimoxazole be discontinued:

- Occurrence of severe cutaneous reactions such as Stevens Johnson syndrome, renal and/or hepatic insufficiency or severe hematological toxicity.
- In an HIV exposed child ONLY once HIV infection has confidently been excluded;
- For a non-breastfeeding child <18 months of age this is by negative DNA or RNA virological HIV testing
- For a breastfed HIV exposed child < 18months-negative virological testing is only reliable if conducted 6 weeks after cessation of breastfeeding,
- For a breastfed HIV-exposed child >18 months-negative HIV antibody testing 3 months after stopping breastfeeding
- In an HIV-infected child:
- If the child is on ARV therapy, cotrimoxazole can be stopped ONLY when evidence of immune restoration has occurred. This can be assumed where the child is over 18 months of age and CD4% 15 at two measurements, at least 3 to 6 months apart. If a CD4

count is not available, cotrimoxazole should not be stopped before a full 6 months of successful adherence to ARV therapy, and then only when clinical evidence of immune restoration is present.

- Continuing cotrimoxazole may continue to provide benefit even once child has clinically improved.
- If ARV therapy is not available it should not be discontinued

What doses of cotrimoxazole should be used?

- Syrup use is recommended in very young children up to 10-12 kg
- Recommended dosages of 6-8 mg/kg once daily should be used.
- Once tablets can be taken, half of a standard adult tablet crushed may be used for children up to 10kg, one whole tablet for 10-25kg, two single strength or one double strength for over 25kg (a usual single strength tablet provides Sulfamethoxazole 400 mg and trimethoprim 80 mg).
- Use weight band dosages rather than body surface area doses
- If the child is allergic to cotrimoxazole, dapsone is the best alternative

What follow-up is required?

- Assessment of tolerance and adherence: Cotrimoxazole prophylaxis should be a routine part of care of HIV infected children, and be assessed at all regular clinic visits or follow-up visits by health workers and/or other members of multidisciplinary care teams.
- Initial clinic follow-up in children is suggested monthly, and then every three months, if cotrimoxazole is well tolerated.

## Other Operational Issues

### *Drug Supplies*

- Cotrimoxazole should be prescribed by the health care providers responsible for HIV care of the child.

- Providers should ensure regular sustained supply of high quality cotrimoxazole, and ensure the child has enough supply until after the next scheduled appointment for regular monitoring or ARV related care. This should ensure doses are not missed.
- Governments need to ensure an uninterrupted drug supply for both treatment and prophylaxis is available. This requires accurately estimating programme needs and extra budgetary allocation.
- Existing drug distribution systems should be used for supply
- Private sector including industry and other medical insurance plans, should be encouraged to provide prophylaxis to families and include provision for children

## Patient Information

Patients need to be clear that while cotrimoxazole does not cure HIV, regular dosing is essential for protection of children from infections that are more common or more likely to occur in HIV infection. Cotrimoxazole does not replace the need for antiretroviral therapy.

## Policy and Programme Information

- National AIDS treatment, care and support policies and strategies include provision of cotrimoxazole prophylaxis
- National ARV treatment guidelines, PMTCT guidelines, and clinical care guidelines include cotrimoxazole prophylaxis for HIV exposed and HIV infected children
- Health providers at all levels are sensitized and trained to provide cotrimoxazole prophylaxis to all HIV-exposed and HIV-infected children
- Countries should supply the cotrimoxazole for children free of charge or at subsidized rates where possible Monitoring and evaluation

In order to monitor progress towards the delivery of comprehensive AIDS treatment, care and support, National programmes should assess the extent to which the range of

HIV related care services are being implemented and set clear targets for children. Cotrimoxazole prophylaxis is an essential health intervention that needs to be included in child health services (including IMCI), PMTCT services, TB services and HIV ART treatment services (facility based and community based). Monitoring of progress towards achieving this should include:

- Monitoring the provision of cotrimoxazole prophylaxis to children and adolescents within existing care services (including, paediatric HIV care, home based care and IMCI).
- Documenting the proportion of HIV-exposed infants in PMTCT programs who receive cotrimoxazole interventions until confirmation of HIV infection status.
- National monitoring of antimicrobial resistance of pneumonia, dysentery and malaria in children is recommended because cotrimoxazole is widely used for other clinical indications.

## GLOBAL AIDS-INDIA

India's HIV positive children to get free drugs-Sushma makes a promise which will cost ministry thrice its budget.

New Delhi report-October 4, 2003-TOUFIQ RASHID

The Government is embarking on an ambitious project to provide anti-retroviral drugs to HIV-positive children below 14 years of age free of cost. This will enhance their life and help them fight the virus for a long time.

As the non-availability and high cost of the medicines (Rs 5,000 per month) are said to be the major gap in the AIDS control programme in the country, the Government is touting it as a major step forward. The initiative will be included in the next phase of the National Aids Control Organisation (NACO) programme and is likely to start in three-to-six months' time.

It's a huge commitment. Out of the estimated 3.9 to 4.5 million HIV-positive cases in India, around 2 lakh are believed to be children.

And even if half of them need anti-retroviral drugs, the annual spending will be Rs 600 crore. Though the total annual budget of the Health Ministry is just Rs 225 crore, it expects Rs 500 crore global funding and another $100 million from the Bill and Melinda Gates Foundation.

Anti-retroviral drug is the only way an HIV-positive person can live longer. "But most die due to non-availability of the drugs and our major concern is the increasing number of children who contract the illness from their parents. Most of them are orphans or have both parents affected with the virus, so this group was given priority," says Sushma Swaraj, Health and Family Welfare Minister.

Though the Government has no estimates of the budget or the number of people to be covered, it plans to issue a mass appeal for voluntary registration as a first step. "If we hold a survey to estimate the number, it might or might not be conclusive. However, the fact that the medicines would be available for free will help people declare their HIV status to the concerned authorities," the minister says.

According to experts, being HIV-positive doesn't mean that a person is eligible for the anti-retroviral drugs. "A person is given the drugs only when the immunity drops and CD count is below 200," says a NACO official. The state AIDS control organisations have been asked to identify hospitals where the registration can be done.

The minister is meeting the pharma companies next week to discuss the reduction of prices for anti-retroviral drugs in view of the bulk purchase.

# 5

# Hypothesis of HIV/AIDS

According to the oral polio vaccine (OPV) AIDS hypothesis, the AIDS pandemic originated from live polio vaccines prepared in chimpanzee tissue cultures (at least some of which were almost certainly contaminated with chimpanzee SIV) which were administered to up to one million Africans between 1957 and 1960. The specific populations, who may not have been properly informed of the risks before volunteering for the vaccination, were the first in the world to experience HIV-1 infections and AIDS some five to twenty years later.

In particular the experimental oral vaccine, called CHAT, is claimed to have been contaminated with simian immunodeficiency virus (SIV), a group of viruses endemic to African primates and widely accepted as the origin of HIV. Recent evidence shows that CHAT may have been concentrated in African facilities using tissue cultures made from chimpanzee kidneys (more importantly, utilizing chimpanzee serum, containing macrophages, the target of immunodeficiency viruses). Proponents of the OPV AIDS hypothesis include journalist Edward Hooper as well as scientists Louis Paschal and the late W.D. Hamilton.

The OPV AIDS hypothesis is contradicted by a large mass of scientific evidence, and is considered to be incorrect by the scientific community.

## VACCINES

Vaccines are weakened, attenuated versions of pathogens intended to provoke an immune response but not to cause disease. Many vaccines are grown in tissue cultures to increase the concentration of the pathogen and modify its properties. In the 1950s, when the OPV was created, there were no rules about which species to use. Chimpanzee kidneys, in particular, were marked as good cultures for growing polio viruses. Vaccines may be "live" or "killed". Live vaccines contain living pathogens and are more potent than killed vaccines. They provoke a stronger, lasting immune response and usually only one dose is required. However, they are unstable and may be contaminated with unwanted pathogens. In the 1950s, it was common practice to locally amplify oral vaccines, because the concentration of the vaccine changed unpredictably during transport. Although killed polio vaccines had been used with much success, no country wanted to be the first to test a live polio vaccine (Pascal, 1990).

## THE CHAT VACCINE

CHAT was an oral, live experimental vaccine created at the Wistar Institute in Philadelphia by Hilary Koprowski. Between 1957 and 1960 it was given to roughly a million Africans. In Africa, it was administered in the Belgian territories; now the Congo, Rwanda and Burundi.

CHAT was an oral vaccine; it was often squirted from a syringe into the back of the patient's throat. Oral transmission is a proven route for HIV infection. In developing countries, an estimated one-third to one-half of the millions of HIV infected children were infected through breastfeeding. A study comparing oral and rectal exposure of adult macaques to cell-free SIV determined that non traumatic oral exposure was 6000-fold more effective in producing a systemic infection than from rectal exposure. Mucosal cells and oral lesions, as well as the tonsils, are possible entry points for HIV. The vaccine was given to many young infants with undeveloped immune systems. In Africa, it was standard to transport a small amount of the original vaccine and then locally amplify it using local facilities and tissue cultures harvested from native animals. In South Africa, African green monkey tissue was used to amplify the Sabin vaccine. In French West Africa and Equatorial Africa, baboons were used to amplify a vaccine from the Pasteur Institute. And in Poland, the CHAT vaccine was amplified using Asian macaques.

## RECENT DISCOVERIES

In 2003, Edward Hooper and colleagues travelled to the Democratic Republic of Congo and uncovered testimony supporting the OPV hypothesis. In the Congo, the Laboratoire Medical de Stanleyville (LMS) was responsible for testing the CHAT vaccine and performing the initial set of vaccinations. A few miles from LMS was Lindi Camp, a chimpanzee colony at which more than 500 chimps and bonobos, collected from a 300km radius, were sacrificed between 1956 and 1960.

In Kisangani, Hooper talked to former lab technicians that had worked on the vaccination program at LMS. Jacques Kanyama, a virology technician, alleged that batches of CHAT had been prepared locally, a possibility formerly denied by Belgian and American staff who claimed that the lab was too primitive and lacked equipment. According to Kanyama, Paul Osterrieth, in charge of the virology department, had been producing an oral polio vaccine on-site. Philip Elebe, a microbiology technician, claimed that tissue cultures were being produced from Lindi chimpanzees. Osterrieth disputes these claims, saying that no vaccine was prepared locally and that only the CHAT vaccine from America was used. If the accounts are true, they describe a clear mechanism for the introduction of HIV into the human population.

## HISTORY

In 1987 Louis Pascal began to suspect that polio vaccines contaminated with SIVs could be responsible for the AIDS epidemic. By reading medical journals from the 1950s and 1960s and comparing with what was known about the first cases of HIV infection, he concluded that Koprowski's CHAT Type 1 vaccine administered in Belgian Congo between 1957 and 1960 was a likely source.

In the same year Blaine Elswood, an AIDS treatment activist who had developed similar ideas, contacted the journalist Tom Curtis about a "bombshell story." Curtis investigated the story and published an article in Rolling Stone 1992.. Hilary Koprowski sued the Rolling Stone and Tom Curtis for defamation. The magazine published a "retraction" which praised Dr. Koprowski and absolved him from any blame for the introduction of AIDS to the human population: "we never wished to suggest that it has been scientifically proven that Koprowski is the father of AIDS." However the "retraction" also reiterated that the OPV theory was "one of several disputed and unproven theories". Rolling Stone had to pay $US 1 in damages and around $US 500,000 for legal fees. The legal action cost Dr Koprowski around $US 300,000.

A few scientists, notably the biologist W.D. Hamilton thought the theory required serious investigation, but they received little support from the scientific community. Hamilton wrote a letter to Science in 1994 supporting Pascal and Curtis, but it was rejected by the editors. Journalist Edward Hooper, who had already begun to investigate the origin of AIDS when the OPV theory was first put forward gradually became convinced of its truth. After nine years of investigations, he detailed the theory and evidence in his 1999 book, The River. In 2004, the Origin of Aids, a TV documentary strongly supportive of the OPV theory, appeared on television stations globally.

**CRITICISM**

For 15 years, the OPV AIDS theory has been criticized by members of the scientific and medical establishment as being unfounded, unlikely or inconsistent with HIV epidemiology. However, although these criticisms are widely publicized, particularly by mainstream science journals, some people remain convinced of the OPV hypothesis and controversy continues. In October 1992, the journal Science ran a story titled "Panel Nixes Congo Vaccine as AIDS source," on the basis of a panel arranged by the Wistar Institute, an organization at the center of this controversy. In September 2000, 6 samples of the CHAT vaccine from the Wistar Institute were independently tested and no trace of HIV, SIV or chimpanzee DNA was found. This led to widespread announcements of the death of the OPV theory, for example Robin Weiss's article in Nature titled 'Polio vaccines exonerated.' But the samples were not from the same batch as was given out in Kinshasa.

However, in April 2004, claims by the OPV AIDS theory that Kisangani chimpanzees were, indirectly, the true source of HIV-1 was finally put to rest by an article which appeared in Nature entitled "Origin of AIDS: contaminated polio vaccine theory refuted." In the article, researchers Michael Worobey and colleagues verified the existence of SIVcpz in Kisangani chimps. However, through phylogenetic analyzes of the virus, they found the SIVcpz that infected these chimps was nested within an entirely different clade of SIVcpz than the strain that includes HIV-1. These results show that the Kisangani chimpanzees could not have been the source of HIV-1. Further, the article proclaims the disproval of a central tenet to the OPV AIDS theory. Hooper disputes this proclamation by asserting the OPV theory never completely relied on the now disproven premise. He explains OPV chimpanzees came from other areas as well.

Critics claim that the OPV hypothesis, if widely known, would undermine public confidence in mass vaccination programs and, in particular, UN plans to eradicate polio. Some, such as Hilary Koprowski, have claimed that anti-vaccine sentiment in Africa has intensified due to the publicization of the hypothesis. However, Hooper argues that conspiratorial rumours about vaccination have been prevalent for most of the century and do not relate to the OPV hypothesis. Hooper also points out that he does not claim that modern polio vaccines are anything but safe.

## THE SV40

If polio vaccination were responsible for AIDS, it would not be without precedent. SV40, the 40th discovered simian virus, was introduced into the human population in the 1950s by contaminated polio vaccines produced in Asian rhesus monkey kidney cells. It now infects some humans, although it is unclear if it can be passed by human-to-human contact. Research has shown that SV40 induces tumours in hamsters, and has been found present in human brain tumors, mesotheliomas and bone tumors. There is some evidence that SV40 exposure could lead to cancer in humans under natural conditions, but the evidence is far from conclusive.

A similar case occurred in 1942, in which 50,000 US servicemen were infected with acute hepatitis B due to contaminated yellow fever vaccine.

## ZOONOSES

A zoonosis is a disease capable of passing between animals and humans. Like other AIDS origin hypotheses, the OPV hypothesis depends on zoonotic transfer to explain the spread of SIV into the human population and its evolution into HIV. Examples of zoonotic transfer include Ebola virus, Marburg virus and SV40. Arguments against xenotransplantation, the transfer of animal tissue into humans, are supported by the OPV hypothesis, if proven. Such medical experimentation could lead to future epidemics of unknown animal viruses and prions.

## AIDS REAPPRAISAL

The AIDS reappraisal movement or AIDS dissident movement, pejoratively referred to as AIDS denialism, is a loosely connected group of activists, journalists, scientists, and HIV-positive persons who dispute the scientific consensus that the human immunodeficiency virus (HIV) is the cause of acquired immune deficiency syndrome (AIDS). Dissidents argue that the consensus that HIV causes AIDS has resulted in inaccurate diagnoses, psychological terror, toxic treatments, and a squandering of public funds, as well as an unprecedented deviation from scientific method and standards.

The majority of the scientific community considers the causative role of HIV to be proven; dissident arguments are felt to be the result of cherry-picking of predominantly outdated scientific data, with the potential to endanger public health by dissuading people from utilizing proven treatments.

## A BRIEF HISTORY

- *1983:* A group of scientists and doctors at the Pasteur Institute in France, led by Luc Montagnier, discovers a new virus in a patient with signs and symptoms that often precede AIDS. They name their discovery lymphadenopathy-associated virus, or LAV, and send samples to Robert Gallo's team in the United States.
- *1984:* On April 23, at a Washington press conference held two weeks before the relevant papers are published, Margaret Heckler, then Secretary of Health and Human

Services, announces that Gallo and his co-workers have discovered a virus that is the "probable" cause of AIDS. This virus is initially named HTLV-III.

- *1984:* Casper Schmidt responds to the publication of Gallo's papers by writing "The Group-Fantasy Origins of AIDS", which is published by the Journal of Psychohistory. He posits that AIDS is an example of "epidemic hysteria" in which groups of people are subconsciously acting out social conflicts, and compares it to documented cases of epidemic hysteria in the past which were mistakenly thought to be infectious.
- *1986:* The viruses discovered by Montagnier and Gallo, having been found to be genetically indistinguishable, are renamed HIV.
- *1987:* Peter Duesberg questions the HIV theory of AIDS for the first time in his paper "Retroviruses as Carcinogens and Pathogens: Expectations and Reality", published in the journal Cancer Research. This publication coincides with the start of major public health campaigns and the promotion of AZT as a treatment.
- *1988:* The Perth Group, led by Eleni Papadopulos-Eleopulos, publishes their first article questioning aspects of the mainstream ideas about HIV and AIDS. They conclude that there is "no compelling reason for preferring the viral hypothesis of AIDS to one based on the activity of oxidising agents."
- *1990:* Robert Root-Bernstein publishes his first peer-reviewed article detailing his objections to the mainstream view of AIDS and HIV, entitled "Do we know the cause(s) of AIDS?" In it, he questions both the mainstream view and the dissident view as potentially inaccurate.
- *1991:* The Group for the Scientific Reappraisal of the HIV-AIDS Hypothesis, comprised of twelve scientists, doctors, and activists, submits a short letter to various journals. Another similar letter would be published 4 years later in the journal Science.

- *1994, 28 October:* Robert Willner, a physician whose medical license was revoked for, among other things, treating an AIDS patient with ozone therapy, publicly jabs his finger with blood he says is from an HIV-infected patient. Willner died the following year of a heart attack.
- *1995:* The dissident group Continuum places an advertisement in The Pink Paper offering a £1,000 reward to "the first person finding one scientific paper establishing actual isolation of HIV" (according to their specific set of rules).
- *1996:* Various scientists, including Duesberg, dismiss the Continuum challenge, asserting that HIV doubtlessly exists.
- *2000:* South Africa's President, Thabo Mbeki, invites several dissidents to join his Presidential AIDS Advisory Panel. The scientific community responds with the Durban declaration, a document affirming that HIV causes AIDS, signed by over 5,000 scientists and physicians.
- *2006:* Celia Farber, a journalist and prominent AIDS dissident, publishes an essay in the March issue of Harper's entitled Out of Control: AIDS and the Corruption of Medical Science, in which she summarizes a number of arguments for AIDS reappraisal and alleges incompetence, conspiracy, and fraud on the part of the mainstream medical community.
- *2007:* South African advocate Anthony Brink serves a file of indictment at the International Criminal Court against Zackie Achmat and the Treatment Action Campaign (TAC), charging that their efforts to expand access to antiretroviral medication in South Africa constitute "genocide", and suggesting that Achmat be locked in "a small white steel and concrete cage" and "eradicated". The TAC responds by describing the indictment as "truly delusional".

## THE AIDS DISSIDENT COMMUNITY

People critical of the mainstream view of AIDS include HIV-positive persons, government employees, scientists, doctors and activists in several countries. Probably the most famous and influential AIDS dissident scientist is Peter Duesberg, professor of molecular and cell biology at the University of California, Berkeley, who has been contesting the mainstream view of AIDS causation since 1987. Other scientists include David Rasnick (who has patents on protease inhibitors used in the treatment of AIDS) and Rodney Richards (who helped to develop some of the first commercial HIV antibody tests). Nobel Prize winner Kary Mullis, inventor of PCR, has expressed sympathy for dissident theories.

Some prominent AIDS dissidents, such as Tom Bethell and Phillip E. Johnson, have expressed support for a wide range of controversial or pseudoscientific beliefs, including intelligent design and global warming skepticism.

Other notable AIDS dissidents include Australian academic Hiram Caton, journalist Celia Farber and activist Christine Maggiore. Nate Mendel, bassist with the rock band Foo Fighters, has expressed support for AIDS dissident ideas and organized a benefit concert in January 2000 for the AIDS dissident organization Alive & Well AIDS Alternatives.

Organizations of AIDS dissidents include the Perth Group and the Group for the Scientific Reappraisal of the HIV-AIDS Hypothesis.

## FORMER DISSIDENTS

Several prominent figures once associated with AIDS reappraisal have since changed their views and accepted that HIV plays a role in causing AIDS, in response to an accumulation of newer studies and data. Robert Root-Bernstein, author of Rethinking AIDS: The Tragic Cost of Premature Consensus and formerly a critic of the HIV/AIDS paradigm, has since distanced himself from the AIDS dissident movement, saying, "The denialists make claims that are clearly inconsistent with existing studies. When I check the existing studies, I don't agree with the interpretation of the data, or, worse, I can't find the studies [at all]." In a 2005 article, Root-Bernstein and his coauthor wrote that, "It is well-known that HIV-1 infection results in a gradual decline of the CD4+ T-lymphocytes."

Joseph Sonnabend, who until the late 1990s regarded the issue of AIDS causation as unresolved, has reconsidered in light of the success of newer antiretroviral drugs, stating, "The evidence now strongly supports a role for HIV... Drugs that can save your life can also under different circumstances kill you. This is a distinction that denialists do not seem to understand."

Both Sonnabend and Root-Bernstein now favor a less controversial hypothesis, suggesting that cofactors in addition to HIV are necessary to cause AIDS. Nonetheless, as of November 2006, some dissident websites continue to claim that Root-Bernstein and Sonnabend deny the role of HIV in AIDS.

## POINTS OF CONTENTION

Although members of the AIDS dissident community are united by their disagreement with the concept that HIV is the cause of AIDS, the specific positions taken by various groups differ.

Dissident arguments have centered around claims that HIV does not exist or has not been adequately isolated, that the virus does not fulfill Koch's postulates, that HIV testing is inaccurate, or that antibodies to HIV neutralize the virus and render it harmless. Suggested alternative causes of AIDS include recreational drugs, malnutrition and the very antiretroviral drugs used to treat the syndrome.

Such claims have been examined extensively in the peer-reviewed medical and scientific literature; a scientific consensus has arisen that dissident claims have been convincingly disproved, and that HIV does indeed cause AIDS. Accumulating evidence of the significant benefits of modern anti-HIV medication are seen as further confirmation of HIV's role in AIDS.

# 6

# The Disease Staging System for HIV: WHO Programme

WHO Disease Staging System for HIV Infection and Disease was first produced in 1990 by the World Health Organisation and updated in September 2005. It is an approach for use in resource limited settings and is widely used in Africa and Asia and has been a useful research tool in studies of progression to symptomatic HIV disease. Most of these conditions are opportunistic infections that can be easily treated in healthy people. The staging system is different for adults and adolescents and children.

**Stage I:** HIV disease is asymptomatic and not categorized as AIDS.

**Stage II:** Include minor mucocutaneous manifestations and recurrent upper respiratory tract infections.

**Stage III:** Includes unexplained chronic diarrhea for longer than a month, severe bacterial infections and pulmonary tuberculosis.

**Stage IV:** Includes toxoplasmosis of the brain, candidiasis of the esophagus, trachea, bronchi or lungs and Kaposi's sarcoma; these diseases are used as indicators of AIDS.

## DISEASE IN ADULTS AND ADOLESCENTS

WHO Disease Staging System for HIV Infection and Disease in Adults and Adolescents was first produced in 1990 by the World Health Organization and updated in September 2005. It is an approach for use in resource limited settings and is widely used in Africa and Asia and has been a useful research tool in studies of progression to symptomatic HIV disease. Following infection with HIV, the rate of clinical disease progression varies enormously between individuals. Many factors such as host susceptibility and immune function, health care and co-infections, as well as factors relating to the viral strain may affect the rate of clinical disease progression. Revised World Health Organization (WHO) Clinical Staging of HIV/ AIDS For Adults and Adolescents (2005) (This is the interim African Region version for persons aged 15 years or more who have had a positive HIV antibody test or other laboratory evidence of HIV infection) (It must be noted that the UN defines adolescents as persons aged 10-19 years but for surveillance purposes, the category of adults and adolescents comprises people aged 15 years and over)

**Primary HIV Infection:**

- Asymptomatic
- Acute retroviral syndrome

**Clinical Stage 1:**

- Asymptomatic
- Persistent generalized lymphadenopathy

**Clinical Stage 2:**

- Moderate and unexplained weight loss (<10% of presumed or measured body weight)
- Recurrent respiratory tract infections (such as sinusitis, bronchitis, otitis media, pharyngitis)
- Herpes zoster
- Recurrent oral ulcerations
- Papular pruritic eruptions
- Angular cheilitis
- Seborrhoeic dermatitis
- Fungal finger nail infections

**Clinical Stage 3:** Conditions where a presumptive diagnosis can be made on the basis of clinical signs or simple investigations:

- Unexplained chronic diarrhoea for longer than one month

- Unexplained persistent fever (intermittent or constant for longer than one month)
- Severe weight loss (>10% of presumed or measured body weight)
- Oral candidiasis
- Oral hairy leukoplakia
- Pulmonary tuberculosis (TB) diagnosed in last two years
- Severe presumed bacterial infections (e.g. pneumonia, empyema, meningitis, bacteraemia, pyomyositis, bone or joint infection)
- Acute necrotizing ulcerative stomatitis, gingivitis or periodontitis

**Conditions where Confirmatory Diagnostic Testing is Necessary:**

- Unexplained anaemia (< 80 g/l), and or neutropenia (<500/μl) and or thrombocytopenia (<50 000/μl) for more than one month

**Clinical Stage 4:** Conditions where a presumptive diagnosis can be made on the basis of clinical signs or simple investigations

- HIV wasting syndrome
- Pneumocystis pneumonia
- Recurrent severe or radiological bacterial pneumonia
- Chronic herpes simplex infection (orolabial, genital or anorectal of more than one month's duration)
- Oesophageal candidiasis
- Extrapulmonary Tuberculosis
- Kaposi's sarcoma
- Central nervous system toxoplasmosis
- HIV encephalopathy

**Conditions where Confirmatory Diagnostic Testing is Necessary:**

- Extrapulmonary cryptococcosis including meningitis
- Disseminated non-tuberculous mycobacteria infection

- Progressive multifocal leukoencephalopathy
- Candida of trachea, bronchi or lungs
- Cryptosporidiosis
- Isosporiasis
- Visceral herpes simplex infection
- Cytomegalovirus (CMV) infection (retinitis or of an organ other than liver, spleen or lymph nodes)
- Any disseminated mycosis (e.g. histoplasmosis, coccidiomycosis, penicilliosis)
- Recurrent non-typhoidal salmonella septicaemia
- Lymphoma (cerebral or B cell non-Hodgkin)
- Invasive cervical carcinoma
- Visceral leishmaniasis

**Original proposal in 1990**

**Clinical Stage I:**

- Asymptomatic
- Generalised lymphadenopathy

**Performance Scale:** 1: asymptomatic, normal activity.

**Clinical Stage II:**

- Weight loss, < 10% of body weight
- Minor mucocutaneous manifestations (seborrheic dermatitis, prurigo, fungal nail infections, recurrent oral ulcerations, angular cheilitis)
- Herpes zoster within the last five years
- Recurrent upper respiratory tract infections (i.e. bacterial sinusitis)

**And/or Performance Scale 2:** Symptomatic, normal activity.

**Clinical Stage III:**

- Weight loss, > 10% of body weight
- Unexplained chronic diarrhoea > 1 month

- Unexplained prolonged fever (intermittent or constant), > 1 month
- Oral [candidiasis] ([thrush])
- Oral hairy leucoplakia
- Pulmonary tuberculosis
- Severe bacterial infections (i.e. pneumonia, pyomyositis)

And/or performance scale 3: bedridden < 50% of the day during last month.

**Clinical Stage IV:** The declaration of AIDS:

- HIV wasting syndrome
- Pneumocystis carinii pneumonia
- Toxoplasmosis of the brain
- Cryptosporidiosis with diarrhoea > 1 month
- Cryptococcosis, extrapulmonary
- Cytomegalovirus disease of an organ other than liver, spleen or lymph node (ex: retinitis)
- Herpes simplex virus infection, mucocutaneous (>1 month) or visceral
- Progressive multifocal leucoencephalopathy
- Any disseminated endemic mycosis
- Candidiasis of esophagus, trachea, bronchi
- Atypical mycobacteriosis, disseminated or lungs
- Non-typhoid Salmonella septicemia
- Extrapulmonary tuberculosis
- Lymphoma
- Kaposi's sarcoma
- HIV encephalopathy?

And/or performance scale 4: bedridden > 50% of the day during last month.

(*) HIV wasting syndrome: weight loss of > 10% of body weight, plus either unexplained chronic diarrhoea (> 1 month) or chronic weakness and unexplained prolonged fever (> 1 month).

(?)HIV encephalopathy: clinical findings of disabling cognitive and/or motor dysfunction interfering with activities of daily living, progressing over weeks to months, in the absence of a concurrent illness or condition other than HIV infection which could explain the findings.

## AIDS DEMENTIA COMPLEX

AIDS dementia complex (ADC; also known as HIV dementia, HIV encephalopathy and HIV-associated dementia) has become a common neurological disorder associated with HIV infection and AIDS. It is a metabolic encephalopathy induced by HIV infection and fueled by immune activation of brain macrophages and microglia. These cells are actively infected with HIV and secrete neurotoxins of both host and viral origin. The essential features of ADC are disabling cognitive impairment accompanied by motor dysfunction, speech problems and behavioural change. Cognitive impairment is characterised by mental slowness, trouble with memory and poor concentration. Motor symptoms include a loss of fine motor control leading to clumsiness, poor balance and tremors. Behavioural changes may include apathy, lethargy and diminished emotional responses and spontaneity. Histopathologically, it is identified by the infiltration of monocytes and macrophages into the central nervous system (CNS), gliosis, pallor of myelin sheaths, abnormalities of dendritic processes and neuronal apoptosis.

ADC typically occurs after years of HIV infection and is associated with low CD4+ T cell levels and high plasma viral loads. It is sometimes seen as the first sign of the onset of AIDS. Prevalence is between 10-20% in Western countries and has only been seen in 1-2% of India based infections. With the advent of highly active antiretroviral therapy (HAART), the frequency of ADC has declined in developed countries. HAART may not only prevent or delay the onset of ADC in people with HIV infection, it can also improve mental function in people who already have ADC.

Dementia only exists when neurocognitive impairment in the patient is severe enough to interfere markedly with day-to-day function. That is, the patient is typically unable to work and may not be able to take care of him or herself. Before this, the patient is said to have a mild neurocognitive disorder.

## Diagnostic Criteria

1. Marked acquired impairment of at least two ability domains of cognitive function (e.g. memory, attention): typically, the impairment is in multiple domains, especially in learning, information processing and concentration/attention. The cognitive impairment is ascertained by medical history, mental status examination or neuropsychological testing.
2. Cognitive impairments identified in 1. interfere markedly with day-to-day functioning.
3. Cognitive impairments identified in 1. are present for at least one month.
4. Cognitive impairments identified in 1. do not meet the criteria for delirium, or if delirium is present, dementia was diagnosed when delirium was not present.
5. No evidence of another, pre-existing aetiology that could explain the dementia (e.g. another CNS infection, CNS neoplasm, cerebrovascular disease, pre-existing neurological disease, severe substance abuse compatible with CNS disorder.

While the progression of dysfunction is variable, it is regarded as a serious complication and, untreated, can progress to a fatal outcome. Diagnosis is made by neurologists who carefully rule out alternative diagnoses. This routinely requires a careful neurological examination, brain scans (MRI or CT scan) and a lumbar puncture to evaluate the cerebrospinal fluid.

No single test is available to confirm the diagnosis, but the constellation of history, laboratory findings, and examination can reliably establish the diagnosis when performed by experienced clinicians. The amount of virus in the brain does not correlate well with the degree of dementia, suggesting that secondary mechanisms are also important in the manifestation of ADC.

## RESEARCH

AIDS Dementia Complex (ADC) is not a true opportunistic infection. It is one of the few conditions caused directly by HIV itself. But it is not quite as simple as that because the central nervous system can be damaged by a number of other causes:

- opportunistic infections-there are many
- Primary cerebral lymphoma or metastasis of other AIDS-related cancers
- direct effects of HIV in the brain
- toxic effects of drug treatments
- malnutrition

Many researchers believe that HIV damages the vital brain cells, neurons, indirectly. According to one theory, HIV either infects or activates cells that nurture and maintain the brain, known as macrophages and microglia. These cells then produce toxins that can set off a series of reactions that instruct neurons to kill themselves. The infected macrophages and microglia also appear to produce additional factors chemokines and cytokines-that can affect neurons as well as other brain cells known as astrocytes. The affected astrocytes, which normally nurture and protect neurons, also may now end up harming neurons. Researchers hope that new drugs under investigation will interfere with the detrimental cycle and prevent neuron death.

## ADC STAGE CHARACTERISTICS

- Stage 0 (Normal) Normal Mental and Motor Function
- Stage 0.5 (Subclinical) Minimal symptoms of cognitive or motor dysfunction characteristic of ADC, or mild signs (snout response, slowed extremity movements), but without impairment of work or capacity to perform activities of daily living (ADL). Gait and strength are normal.
- Stage 1 (Mild) Evidence of functional intellectual or motor impairment characteristic of ADC, but able to perform all but the more demanding aspects of work or ADL. Can walk without assistance.

- Stage 2 (Moderate) Cannot work or maintain the more demanding aspects of daily life, but able to perform basic activities of self care. Ambulatory, but may require a single prop.
- Stage 3 (Severe) Major intellectual incapacity-cannot follow news or personal events, cannot sustain complex conversation, considerable slowing of all output. And/ or motor disability-cannot walk unassisted, requiring walker or personal support, usually with slowing and clumsiness of arms as well.
- Stage 4 (End Stage) Nearly vegetative. Intellectual and social comprehension and responses are at a rudimentary level. Nearly or absolutely mute. Paraparetic or paraplegic with double incontinence

## ANTIRETROVIRAL DRUG

Antiretroviral drugs are medications for the treatment of infection by retroviruses, primarily HIV. Different classes of antiretroviral drugs act at different stages of the HIV life cycle. Combination of several (typically three or four) antiretroviral drugs is known as Highly Active Anti-Retroviral Therapy (HAART).

Organizations such as the National Institutes of Health (Bethesda, Maryland, USA) recommend offering antiretroviral treatment to all patients with HIV-related symptoms. However, because of the complexity of selecting and following a regimen, the severity of the side effects, and the importance of compliance to prevent viral resistance, such organizations emphasize the importance of involving patients in therapy choices and recommend analyzing the risks and the potential benefits to patients without symptoms.

### Classes of Antiretroviral Drugs

Antiretroviral drugs are broadly classified by the phase of the retrovirus life-cyle that the drug inhibits. There are thus five broad classifications of antiretroviral drugs in development, though only the first three classes currently have licensed examples:

- Reverse transcriptase inhibitors (RTIs) target construction of viral DNA by inhibiting activity of reverse transcriptase. There are two subtypes of RTIs with different mechanisms of action: nucleoside-analogue RTIs are incorporated into the viral DNA leading to chain termination, while non-nucleoside-analogue RTIs distort the binding potential of the reverse transcriptase enzyme.
- Protease inhibitors (PIs) target viral assembly by inhibiting the activity of protease, an enzyme used by HIV to cleave nascent proteins for final assembly of new virons.
- Fusion inhibitors block HIV from fusing with a cell's membrane to enter and infect it. (There is currently only one FDA-approved drug in this class, enfuvirtide, marketed as Fuzeon.)
- Integrase inhibitors inhibit the enzyme integrase, which is responsible for integration of viral DNA into the DNA of the infected cell. (There are several integrase inhibitors currently under clinical trial but none are commercially available.)
- Entry inhibitors block HIV-1 from the host cell by binding CCR5, a molecule on the viral membrane termed a co-receptor that HIV-1 normally uses for entry into the cell.

**Fixed dose Combinations**

Fixed dose combinations are multiple antiretroviral drugs combined into a single pill.

**Synergistic Enhancers**

Synergistic enhancers either do not possess antiretroviral properties alone or are inadequate or impractical for monotherapy, but when they are taken concurrently with antiretroviral drugs they enhance the effect of that drug (often by altering the metabolism of the other antiretroviral). These include ritonavir. Ritonavir is per se an antiretroviral drug which belongs to the class of protease inhibitors. It can however be administered at a "baby" dosage to reduce the liver metabolism of other antiretroviral drugs. This principle was first exploited in the drug Kaletra (Abbott), which is a combination of ritonavir with the protease inhibitor lopinavir at a ratio (v/v) of 1:5. Ritonavir is also used as an enhancer of other protease inhibitors such as saquinavir and atazanavir, and of the investigational integrase inhibitor, GS-9137. Other synergistic enhancers are being investigated for this purpose.

### Combination Therapy

The life cycle of HIV can be as short as about 1.5 days: from viral entry into a cell; through replication, assembly, and release of additional viruses; to infection of other cells. HIV lacks proofreading enzymes to correct errors made when it converts its RNA into DNA via reverse transcription. Its short life cycle and high error rate cause the virus to mutate very rapidly, resulting in a high genetic variability of HIV. Most of the mutations either are inferior to the parent virus (often lacking the ability to reproduce at all) or convey no advantage, but some of them have a natural selection superiority to their parent and can enable them to slip past defenses such as the human immune system and antiretroviral drugs. The more active copies of the virus, the greater the possibility that one resistant to antiretroviral drugs will be made, so antiretroviral combination therapy defends against resistance by suppressing HIV replication as much as possible.

Combinations of antiretrovirals create multiple obstacles to HIV replication to keep the number of offspring low and reduce the possibility of a superior mutation. If a mutation arises that conveys resistance to one of the drugs being taken, the other drugs continue to suppress reproduction of that mutation. With rare exceptions, no individual antiretroviral drug has been demonstrated to suppress an HIV infection for long; these agents must be taken in combinations in order to have a lasting effect. As a result the standard of care is to use combinations of antiretroviral drugs. Combinations usually comprise two nucleoside-analogue RTIs and one non-nucleoside-analogue RTI or protease inhibitor. Combinations of antiretrovirals are subject to positive and negative synergies, which limits the number of useful combinations. For example, ddI and AZT inhibit each other, so taking them together is less effective than taking either one separately. Other issues further limit some people's treatment options from antiretroviral drug combinations, including their complicated dosing schedules and often severe side effects.

In recent years drug companies have worked together to combine these complex regimens into simpler formulas, termed fixed dose combinations. For instance, two pills containing two or three medications each can be taken twice daily. This greatly increases the ease with which they can be taken, which in turn increases adherence, and thus their effectiveness over long term. Lack of adherence is a primary cause of resistance development in medication-experienced patients. The highly mutanegenic nature of HIV demands 98% adherence to drug cocktails for the drugs to be totally effective (that means missing less than 6 doses per year). Patients able to adhere at this rate and higher can maintain one regimen for up to a decade without developing resistance. This greatly increases chances of long-term survival, as it leaves more drugs available to the patient for longer periods of time.

According to Reference 5 below, "HIV treatment should reduce your viral load to the point at which it is undetectable. An undetectable viral load does not mean that your HIV infection is gone; it simply means that the test is not sensitive enough to detect the small amount of HIV left in your blood," and "Successful HIV treatment can lower your viral load, which may reduce the risk of HIV transmission."

## Current Treatment Guidelines

Antiretroviral drug treatment guidelines have changed many times. Early recommendations attempted a "hit hard, hit early" approach. A more conservative approach followed, with a starting point somewhere between 350 and 500 CD4+ T cells/mm$^3$. The current guidelines use new criteria to consider starting HAART, as described below. However, there remain a range of views on this subject and the decision of whether to commence treatment ultimately rests with the patient and their doctor.

The current guidelines for antiretroviral therapy (ART) from the World Health Organization reflect the 2003 changes to the guidelines and recommend that in resource-limited settings (that is, developing nations), HIV-infected adults and adolescents should start ART when HIV infection has been confirmed and one of the following conditions is present):

- Clinically advanced HIV disease;
- WHO Stage IV HIV disease, irrespective of the CD4 cell count;
- WHO Stage III disease with consideration of using CD4 cell counts less than 350/μl to assist decision making;
- WHO Stage I or II HIV disease with CD4 cell counts less than 200/μl.

The treatment guidelines in the USA are set by the United States Department of Health and Human Services (DHHS). The current guidelines for adults and adolescents were stated on October 6, 2005:

- All patients with history of an AIDS-defining illness or severe symptoms of HIV infection regardless of CD4+ T cell count receive ART.
- Antiretroviral therapy is also recommended for asymptomatic patients with less than 200 CD4+ T cells/μl.
- Asymptomatic patients with CD4+ T cell counts of 201-350 cells/μl should be offered treatment.
- For asymptomatic patients with CD4+ T cell of greater than 350 cells/μl and plasma HIV RNA greater than 100,000 copies/ml, most experienced clinicians defer therapy but some clinicians may consider initiating treatment.
- Therapy should be deferred for patients with CD4+ T cell counts of greater than 350 cells/μl and plasma HIV RNA less than 100,000 copies/mL.

The preferred initial regimens are:

- efavirenz + zidovudine + lamivudine
- efavirenz + tenofovir + emtricitabine

- lopinavir boosted with ritonavir + zidovudine + lamivudine
- lopinavir boosted with ritonavir + tenofovir + emtricitabine.

In countries with a high rate of baseline resistance, resistance testing is recommended prior to starting treatment; or, if the initiation of treatment is urgent, then a "best guess" treatment regimen should be started which is then modified on the basis of resistance testing. In the UK, there is 11.8% medium to high level resistance at baseline to the combination of zidovudine + lamivudine + efavirenz, and 6.4% medium to high level resistance to stavudine + lamivudine + nevirapine.

Because HIV disease progression in children is more rapid than in adults, and laboratory parameters are less predictive of risk for disease progression, particularly for young infants, treatment recommendations from the DHHS have been more aggressive in children than in adults, the current guidelines were published November 3, 2005.

In 2005, the Centers for Disease Control and Prevention in the United States recommended a 28-day HIV drug regimen for those who have been exposed to HIV (HIV Postexposure Prophylaxis [PEP]). The drugs have demonstrated effectiveness in preventing the virus nearly 100% of the time in those who received treatment within the initial 24 hours of exposure. The effectiveness falls to 52% of the time in those who are treated within 72 hours; those not treated within the first 72 hours are not recommended candidates for the regimen.

## CONCERNS

There are several concerns about antiretroviral regimens. The drugs can have serious side effects. Regimens can be complicated, requiring patients to take several pills at various times during the day, although treatment regimens have been greatly simplified in recent years.

If patients miss doses, drug resistance can develop. Also, providing anti-retroviral treatment is costly and resource-intensive, and the majority of the world's infected individuals cannot access treatment services.

Research to improve current treatments includes decreasing side effects of current drugs, further simplifying drug regimens to improve adherence, and determining the best sequence of regimens to manage drug resistance.

**Responses to Treatment in Older Adults**

As people age, their bodies aren't able to repair and rebuild damaged cells, organs or tissues as rapidly as those of younger people. Diseases like HIV that attack and destroy the body's defenses can exacerbate this slowing and increase the risk of developing additional medical problems like diabetes and high blood pressure, and more physical limitations than younger adults with HIV. In the early years of the HIV epidemic (before HAART), older adults' health deteriorated more rapidly than that of younger individuals-regardless of CD4 count. Several studies found that older adults had lower CD4 counts at diagnosis, faster progression to an AIDS diagnosis, more opportunistic infections, and a shorter survival rate than younger adults, regardless of when they were first diagnosed with HIV. Recent studies have found that a person's age doesn't interfere with the ability of HAART to reduce viral load, but there may be differences between younger and older people in how well the immune system responds to treatment. A study published in AIDS (2000) by Roberto Manfredi and Francesco Chiodo examined the effect of HAART on older people (defined as 55 or older) compared to younger people (35 or younger). The study included 21 older people (8 women, 13 men) and 84 younger people (29 women, 55 men). The researchers found that both groups responded to HAART, especially in reducing viral load. However, CD4 counts did not increase as much in the older people relative to the younger ones. On average, CD4 counts increased from 212 to 289 for older adults after one year of HAART. During the same period, CD4 counts rose from 231 to 345 for younger people.

Some people may have a very low CD4 count even though they have an undetectable viral load. This may be related to decreased activity in the thymus (the gland where CD4 cells are made). A 2001 study in AIDS conducted by researchers in Los Angeles included 80 HIV-positive veterans (13 were over 55 and 67 were younger). Although both groups of veterans showed dramatic reductions in viral load once they were on treatment, the researchers found significant differences in CD4 levels at 3, 9, 15, and 18 months. After one year on HAART, average CD4 counts increased by 50 for the older men, compared to increases of 100 for the younger ones. This difference was not related to baseline HIV viral load, coinfection with hepatitis C, or the race/ethnicity of participants. These studies represent an important first step in understanding how their age may affect older adults' response to HIV treatment, but more studies are needed to understand the long-term effects of age on HAART in older adults.

## Limitations of Antiretroviral Drug Therapy

If an HIV infection becomes resistant to standard HAART, there are limited options. One option is to take larger combinations of antiretroviral drugs, an approach known as mega-HAART or salvage therapy. Salvage therapy often increases the drugs' side-effects and treatment costs. Another is to take only one or two antiretroviral drugs, specifically ones that induce HIV mutations that diminish the virulence of the infection. The most common resistance mutation to lamivudine (3TC) in particular appears to do this. Thus, 3TC can be somewhat effective even alone and when the virus is resistant to it. If an HIV infection becomes sufficiently resistant to antiretroviral-drugs, treatment becomes more complicated and prognosis may deteriorate. Treatment options continue to improve as additional new drugs enter clinical trials. However, the limited distribution of many such drugs denies their benefits to patients in the developing world.

Drug holidays (or "structured treatment interruptions"), are intentional discontinuations of antiretroviral drug treatment. Studies of such interruptions attempt to increase the sensitivity of HIV to antiretroviral drugs. The interruptions attempt to change the selection pressure from the drug resistance back toward resistance to the human immune system, thus breeding a more drug-susceptible virus. HIV spends some of its life-cycle in a state where its DNA is entirely integrated into human DNA. Under certain conditions, drug-resistant strains of the virus can remain dormant in this state, since CD4 T-cells also are dormant when not aroused by invading organisms. The resistant strain can then reemerge when antiretroviral drugs are re-introduced.

Intermittent therapy is an experimental approach designed to reduce exposure to antiretroviral drugs in an effort to mitigate side-effects. Intermittent therapy differs from treatment interruptions in that it involves using a much shorter cycle of switching on and off the antiviral drugs. Studies of such approaches include schedules of Week-on, week-off (also known as "wowo") and Five-days-on, two-days-off (also known as "foto"), which skips treatment on weekends. They also seek to determine what kinds of patients are best suited for this approach. However, initial data suggest that intermittent therapy is ineffective and results in drug resistance. It is still unclear whether suppressing or even eliminating HIV will be adequate to restore normal immune function in the long term, since HIV can damage the ability of the thymus to produce normally diverse T-cells. Also, rapid suppression of HIV and partial restoration of the immune system sometimes produces a dangerous hypersensitivity reaction, immune reconstitution inflammatory syndrome. Research continues in these areas.

## Adverse Effects

Adverse effects of antiretroviral drugs vary by drug, by ethnicity, and by individual, and by interaction with other drugs, including alcohol. Hypersensitivity to some drugs may also occur in some individuals. The following list is not complete, but includes several of the common adverse effects experienced by patients taking some antiretroviral drugs:

- Abdominal pain
- Alopecia
- Anemia
- Asthenia
- Diarrhea
- Dizziness (Vertigo)
- Fanconi syndrome
- Flatulence
- Headache

- Hepatitis
- Hyperbilirubinemia
- Hypercholesterolemia (Dyslipidemia, Hyperlipidemia, high cholesterol)
- Hyperpigmentation (of nails, palms, or soles)
- Ingrown nails
- Insomnia
- Jaundice
- Liver failure
- Malaise
- Mental confusion
- Mitochondrial toxicity
- Myalgia
- Myalgic Encephalomyelitis (chronic fatigue syndrome)
- Myopathy
- Nausea
- Neutropenia
- Nightmares
- Oral ulcers
- Pancreatitis
- Paresthesia (numbness)
- Peripheral neuropathy
- Rash
- Renal failure or insufficiency
- Somnolence (drowsiness)
- Stevens-Johnson syndrome
- Change in taste perception
- Vomiting
- Xeroderma (dry skin)
- Xerostomia (dry mouth).

7

# World Societies and Conference of AIDS

The International AIDS Society is the custodian of the International AIDS Conferences, the paramount gathering of all disciplines in HIV/AIDS now held every two years. These prestigious conferences provide a unique forum for the interaction of science, community and leadership with the goal of bringing knowledge together for changes in the world's response to HIV/AIDS. These conferences started in 1985 in Atlanta, Georgia, USA. They were held annually until 1994 when they became biennial. Below is the list of conferences and their venue:

| Year | Number | Venue | Theme |
|---|---|---|---|
| 1985 | I | Atlanta, GA, USA | none |
| 1986 | II | Paris, France | none |
| 1987 | III | Washington, D.C., USA | none |
| 1988 | IV | Stockholm, Sweden | none |
| 1989 | V | Montréal, Canada | The Scientific and Social Challenge of AIDS |
| 1990 | VI | San Francisco, CA, USA | AIDS in the Nineties: From Science to Policy |
| 1991 | VII | Florence, Italy | Science Challenging AIDS |
| 1992 | VIII | Amsterdam, The Netherlands | A World United Against AIDS |
| 1993 | IX | Berlin, Germany | none |
| 1994 | X | Yokohama, Japan | The Global Challenge of AIDS: Together for the future |

*Contd...*

| Year | Number | Venue | Theme |
|---|---|---|---|
| 1996 | XI | Vancouver, Canada | One World One Hope |
| 1998 | XII | Geneva, Switzerland | Bridging the Gap (Conference website) |
| 2000 | XIII | Durban, South Africa | Breaking the Silence |
| 2002 | XIV | Barcelona, Spain | Knowledge and Commitment for Action |
| 2004 | XV | Bangkok, Thailand | Access for All (Conference website) |
| 2006 | XVI | Toronto, Canada | Time to Deliver (Conference website) |

## INTERNATIONAL AIDS SOCIETY

The International AIDS Society (IAS) is the world's professional society for scientists, health care and public health workers, and others engaged in HIV/AIDS prevention, control and care.

The IAS is a non-profit organization founded in 1988. It is politically and financially independent and can speak freely as a voice of reason in AIDS controversies. The IAS president is Pedro Cahn; past presidents have included Helene Gayle, Stephano Vella and Joep Lange. The IAS has more than 10,000 individual members from over 171 countries. The IAS issues a newsletter three times a year and its official journal is AIDS.

The IAS is the custodian of the International AIDS Conference, the paramount gathering of all disciplines in HIV/AIDS. These prestigious conferences were annual between 1985-1994, but are now held every two years. They provide a unique forum for the interaction of science, community and leadership with the goal of bringing knowledge together for changes in the world's response to HIV/AIDS. In 2006, the XVI International AIDS Conference was held in Toronto, Canada. The XVII International AIDS Conference will be held in Mexico City, Mexico from 3-8 August 2008. The IAS also organizes the highly successful IAS Conference on HIV Pathogenesis,

Treatment and Prevention. This conference occurs biennially and focuses solely on the scientific and clinical aspects of HIV/AIDS. It aims to bring together participants from around the world by providing an environment for researchers and clinicians to address current issues in HIV research, prevention and treatment. The IAS 2003 Conference in Paris, France attracted over 6000 delegates from 169 countries. IAS 2005 was held in Rio de Janeiro, Brazil, and IAS 2007 will be held in Sydney, Australia

## PETER PIOT

Dr. Peter Piot (born 1949 in Leuven, Belgium) is Under Secretary-General of the United Nations and Executive Director of the UN specialized agency UNAIDS.

Executive Director of UNAIDS since its creation in 1995 and Under Secretary-General of the United Nations, Dr Peter Piot comes from a distinguished academic and scientific career focusing on AIDS and women's health in the developing world.

Drawing on his skills as a scientist, manager and activist, Dr Piot has challenged world leaders to view AIDS in the context of social and economic development as well as security.

Under his leadership, UN.\IDS has become the chief advocate for worldwide action against AIDS. It has brought together ten organizations of the United Nations system around a common agenda on AIDS, spearheading UN reform.

Dr Piot earned a medical degree from the University of Ghent, a Ph.D. in Microbiology from the University of Antwerp, Belgium, and was a Senior Fellow at the University of Washington in Seattle. After graduating from medical school, Dr Piot co-discovered the Ebola virus in Zaire in 1976.

In the 1980s Dr Piot launched and expanded a series of collaborative projects in Africa-in Burundi, Côte d'Ivoire, Kenya, Tanzania and Zaire. Projet SIDA in Kinshasa, Zaire, was the first international project on AIDS in Africa and is widely acknowledged as having provided the foundations of our understanding of HIV infection in Africa. He was a professor of microbiology, and of public health at the Institute of Tropical Medicine, in Antwerp, and the Universities of Nairobi, Brussels and Lausanne. In 1992, Dr Piot joined the Global Programme on AIDS of the World Health Organization, in Geneva, as Associate Director.

Born in 1949 in Belgium, Dr Piot is fluent in three languages and is the author of 16 books and more than 500 scientific articles. He has received numerous awards for scientific and societal achievement, and was knighted as a Baron by King Albert II of Belgium in 1995. He is a member of the Institute of Medicine of the National Academy of Sciences of the United States and the Royal Academy of Medicine of Belgium, and is a Fellow of the Royal College of Physicians of London, UK.

### Quote, World AIDS Day 2006

The latest global AIDS figures give us reason for concern and for some hope. The number of new infections rose to 4.3 million this year, at the same time 2.9 million people died of AIDS-related illnesses. Multi-drug and extremely drug resistant tuberculosis highlight new challenges in our collective response read more

### Quote, 2006

"On current trends, AIDS will kill tens of millions of people over the next 20 years. But this need not happen. We know prevention works. We know that HIV treatment and care work. The global AIDS response is poised to enter a new era: where leadership and commitment are at long last matched with the resources needed to get on with the job."

## INTERNATIONAL PARTNERSHIP FOR MICROBICIDES

The International Partnership for Microbicides or IPM is a non-profit product development partnership (PDP) established in 2002 to prevent HIV transmission by accelerating the development and availability of a safe and effective microbicide for use by women in developing countries.

## WORLD AIDS DAY

The Red Ribbon is the global symbol for solidarity with HIV-positive people and those living with AIDS.

World AIDS Day, observed December 1 each year, is dedicated to raising awareness of the AIDS pandemic caused by the spread of HIV infection. AIDS has killed more than 25 million people, with an estimated 38.6 million people living with HIV, making it one of the most destructive epidemics in recorded history. Despite recent, improved access to antiretroviral treatment and care in many regions of the world, the AIDS epidemic claimed an estimated 3.1 million (between 2.8 and 3.6 million) lives in 2005 of which, more than half a million (570,000) were children.

The concept of a World AIDS Day originated at the 1988 World Summit of Ministers of Health on Programmes for AIDS Prevention. Since then, it has been taken up by governments, international organizations and charities around the world.

From its inception until 2004, UNAIDS spearheaded the World AIDS Day campaign, choosing annual themes in consultation with other global health organizations. In 2005 this responsibility was turned over to World AIDS Campaign (WAC), who chose Stop AIDS: Keep the Promise as the overarching theme for World AIDS Day observences through 2010, with more specific tag lines chosen annually. This theme is not specific to World AIDS Day, but is used year-round in WAC's efforts to highlight HIV/AIDS within the context of other major global events including the G8 Summit. World AIDS Campaign also conducts "in-country" campaigns throughout the world, like the Student Stop AIDS Campaign, an infection-awareness campaign targeting young people throughout the UK.

***World AIDS Day banner, European Commission building, Brussels***

**World AIDS Day Themes 1988-2010**

| | |
|---|---|
| 1988 | Communication |
| 1989 | Youth |
| 1990 | Women and AIDS |
| 1991 | Sharing the Challenge |
| 1992 | Community Commitment |
| 1993 | Act |

| | |
|---|---|
| 1994 | AIDS and the Family |
| 1995 | Shared Rights, Shared Responsibilities |
| 1996 | One World. One Hope |
| 1997 | Children Living in a World with AIDS |
| 1998 | Force for Change: World AIDS Campaign With Young People |
| 1999 | Listen, Learn, Live: World AIDS Campaign with Children & Young People |
| 2000 | AIDS: Men Make a Difference |
| 2001 | I care. Do you? |
| 2002 | Stigma and Discrimination |
| 2003 | Stigma and Discrimination |
| 2004 | Women, Girls, HIV and AIDS |
| 2005 | Stop AIDS. Keep the Promise |
| 2006 | Stop AIDS. Keep the Promise-Accountability |
| 2007 | Stop AIDS. Keep the Promise |

## TREATMENT ACTION CAMPAIGN

Photo from TAC march on Parliament, Feb 2003-photo from Treatment Action Campaign website.

The Treatment Action Campaign is a South African AIDS activist organization which was founded by the HIV-positive activist Zackie Achmat in 1998. It is unique for combining the issue-specific targeted direct action tactics of North American AIDS groups like ACT UP with the culture and organization of the South African trade union and anti-apartheid movements.

### Founding

The Treatment Action Campaign (TAC) was launched on December 10, 1998, International Human Rights Day. Achmat and a group of ten other activists joined to found the group after anti-apartheid gay rights activist Simon Nkoli died from AIDS even as highly active antiretroviral therapy was available to wealthy South Africans. Shortly thereafter, inspired by the murder of HIV-positive activist Gugu Dlamini, HIV-positive and HIV-negative members of the new group began wearing the group's now-famous T-shirts with the words "HIV Positive" printed boldly in front, a strategy inspired by the apocryphal story of the Danish king wearing the yellow star marking Jews under Nazi occupation. Achmat also became famous for his pledge to not take antiretroviral medicines until all South Africans could obtain them.

Quickly outgrowing its start among a small group of Cape Town activists, TAC became a much more broadly-based group, with chapters in many regions of the nation and a largely black and poor constituency. The group campaigns for greater access to HIV treatment for all South Africans by raising public awareness and understanding about issues surrounding the availability, affordability and use of HIV treatments.

### Suing the Government

The TAC first confronted the South African government for not ensuring that mother-to-child-transmission (MTCT) prevention was available to pregnant mothers. It won this case on the basis of the South African constitutional guarantee of the right to health care, and the government was ordered to provide MTCT programs in public clinics. TAC also assisted the government by defending it in the case brought against the government by the pharmaceutical industry. TAC entered the case as an amicus curiae, submitting a brief in favour of the government's position. Although the withdrawal of the pharmaceutical companies from this case resulted in a government victory, the government showed no interest in providing access to the generic antiretroviral medications that its victory allowed.

Indeed, far from embracing their common victory against the patent rights of multinational companies who were not making affordable drugs available, President Thabo Mbeki began promoting the view that HIV might not cause AIDS and that AIDS medicines were more toxic than helpful, inviting so-called "AIDS dissidents" to advise his government.

### Campaign for Access to Antiretrovirals

Following their legal victories, and facing continuing refusal by the government to make antiretrovirals available, TAC began a campaign for universal access to AIDS treatment through the public health system. In a national congress in 2002, the group decided to confront the government on this issue, first enacting a thousands-strong march on Parliament in February 2003, and then beginning a civil disobedience campaign in March 2003. After assurances from people within the government that a treatment plan would be forthcoming, TAC suspended its civil disobedience campaign. In the summer of 2003, TAC obtained and leaked an internally-circulated government report showing that treatment would be cost-effective because of the likelihood that it would reduce costly hospitalizations within the public-sector health system; however, the government did not endorse the report and condemned the leak. In August 2003, at its next annual congress, TAC voted to resume civil disobedience. TAC members also voted to recommend that Achmat take his medications, which he agreed he would do. At the same time, TAC began a Treatment Project to distribute medications to its activists and to other community members.

Shortly after the Congress, and before the civil disobedience campaign resumed, the Cabinet voted to begin roll-out of antiretroviral access through public-sector health clinics. In the South African system, the Cabinet can overrule the President, and it appeared to have done so in this case.

Although the Cabinet voted to reaffirm that South African AIDS policy is based on the evidence that HIV causes AIDS, President Thabo Mbeki has continued to obliquely suggest support for the denialist position, as has his Minister of Health, Manto Tshabalala-Msimang. The Minister of Health has put special emphasis on nutrition as an alternative to antiretroviral treatment. As the top health official of the nation, she has been a particular target of TAC activism. Although antiretroviral access is now official policy, its implementation has been spotty. TAC continues to protest and sue the government (working with the AIDS Law Project) in order to continue to influence the speed of and approach to the roll-out.

### Successful Legal Challenges to Matthias Rath

Recently, a German vitamin-maker and entrepreneur named Matthias Rath has publicly questioned the effectiveness of HIV medicines in advertisements in South African newspapers. Rath claims that his nutritional products are effective against HIV/AIDS. TAC successfully pursued retractions and corrections from the newspapers, and Rath was censured by the South African media control body. TAC has sued the Minister of Health for failing to stop what it claims are Rath's illegal activities, including "conducting unauthorised experiments on people, distributing unregistered medicines and advertising unproven treatments for AIDS." In a unanimous March 3, 2006 decision, the Cape of Good Hope Provincial Division court found in favour of TAC against Rath in a defamation suit. As a result of this decision, Rath may not claim that TAC is a front for the pharmaceutical industry, a "Trojan horse" or "running dog" of that industry, is funded by the pharmaceutical industry, receives funds from pharmaceutical front organisations in return for promoting antiretroviral medicines, or targets poor communities in order to promote the interests of pharmaceutical companies, since the court found no evidence that any of these allegations were true.

## 2006 IAS Conference and the Global Day of Action

At the XVI International AIDS Society Conference in Toronto, 13-18 August 2006, TAC had a significant presence. Many TAC staff presented in seminars and chaired sessions, most prominently TAC Secretary Sipho Mthathi and Treasurer Mark Heywood. Heywood was a panelist in a plenary session co-chaired by CNN's Sanjay Gupta entitled "Time to Deliver: The Price of Inaction". Towards the end of the session, supporters of TAC, many of whom were wearing the distinctive "HIV POSITIVE" t-shirts, took to the stage behind the panel and silently held placards containing messages such as "Fire Manto", in reference to the Health Minister, who was in attendance. (video). TAC members and supporters also took over the South African government's booth in the exhibitor's area. The booth contained bowls of lemons and garlic, which the Health Minister has claimed contribute to fighting HIV. TAC members passed around these items mockingly, and toyi-toyied inside the booth, attracting attention to the South African government's expenditure on the elaborate booth and lack of corresponding commitment to the national treatment plan. During the conference's closing ceremonies, United Nations Special Envoy for HIV/AIDS in Africa Stephen Lewis pointed out the failure of South Africa's response to HIV/AIDS, calling their actions more "worthy of a lunatic fringe than of a concerned and compassionate state." He also announced that earlier in the morning, Zackie Achmat and 44 others had been arrested for occupying provincial offices in Cape Town in protest of government's failure to treat prisoners with anti-retrovirals, and in particular the recent death of one plaintiff in the legal case against the government on this matter.

After the conclusion of the conference, TAC declared a Global Day of Action for Thursday, August 24, 2006. Protests and marches were held in the U.S., Canada, Brazil, and China by TAC supporters and sympathizers. In South Africa, police used pepper spray on protesters at the Department of Correctional Services building in central Cape Town, though no one was seriously hurt. Similar protests in Gauteng, Eastern Cape, Limpopo, and KwaZulu-Natal were not met with violence. Over 2000 people took part in the demonstrations. The TAC's objective was to deliver its five demands, which include the convening of a national meeting and plan for the HIV/AIDS crisis, the dismissal of the Health Minister, the immediate treatment of prisoners, respect for the rule of law and the Constitution, and the building of a people's health service.

## JOINT UNITED NATIONS PROGRAMME ON HIV/AIDS

The Joint United Nations Programme on HIV and AIDS, or UNAIDS, is the main advocate for accelerated, comprehensive and coordinated global action on the HIV epidemic. UNAIDS' mission is to lead, strengthen and support an expanded response to HIV and AIDS that includes preventing transmission of HIV, providing care and support to those already living with the virus, reducing the vulnerability of individuals and communities to HIV and alleviating the impact of the epidemic.

Five major components make up the role of UNAIDS:

1. Leadership and advocacy for effective action on the epidemic

2. Strategic information and technical support to guide efforts against AIDS worldwide
3. Tracking, monitoring and evaluation of the epidemic and of responses to it
4. Civil society engagement and the development of strategic partnerships
5. Mobilization of resources to support an effective response

Headquartered in Geneva, Switzerland, its first and current executive director is Dr. Peter Piot, Under-Secretary General of the United Nations.

## Governance

UNAIDS is an innovative joint venture of the United Nations (UN) family. UNAIDS brings together the efforts and resources of ten UN system organizations to help the world prevent new HIV infections, care for those already infected, and mitigate the impact of the epidemic.

UNAIDS Cosponsors:

- The Office of the United Nations High Commissioner for Refugees (UNHCR)
- United Nations Children's Fund (UNICEF)
- World Food Programme (WFP)
- United Nations Development Programme (UNDP)
- United Nations Population Fund (UNFPA)
- United Nations Office on Drugs and Crime (UNODC)
- International Labour Organization (ILO)
- United Nations Educational, Scientific and Cultural Organization (UNESCO)
- World Health Organization (WHO)
- World Bank

The Cosponsors and the UNAIDS Secretariat comprise the Committee of Cosponsoring Organizations, which meets annually.

## Role

The aim of UNAIDS is to help mount and support an expanded response-one that engages the efforts of many sectors and partners from government and civil society.

Established in 1994 by a resolution of the UN Economic and Social Council and launched in January 1996, UNAIDS is guided by a Programme Coordinating Board with representatives of 22 governments from all geographic regions, the UNAIDS Cosponsors, and five representatives of nongovernmental organizations (NGOs), including associations of people living with HIV/AIDS.

## Partnerships

The United Nations Declaration Commitment on HIV/AIDS provides the guiding framework for UNAIDS action. Promoting partnerships among various stakeholders is reflected within the leadership section of the Declaration of Commitment. In particular, it calls for complementation of government efforts by the full and active participation of civil society, the business community and the private sector through:

- Establishing and strengthening mechanisms that involve civil society including faith-based organizations (FBOs), the private sector, and people living with HIV/AIDS at all levels
- Encouraging and supporting local and national organizations to expand and strengthen regional partnerships, coalitions and networks
- Full participation of people living with HIV/AIDS (PLWHA), those in vulnerable groups and people mostly at risk, particularly young people
- Addressing issue of stigma and discrimination.

UNAIDS works to promote partnerships among and between this diverse and broad range of non-state entities. This calls for increases in both the number of new actors, as well as in innovative ways of working, to facilitate increased capacity of non-state entities to respond effectively to the epidemic at all levels.

With the momentum generated by the UN Special Session on HIV/AIDS, the main challenges are to:

- Sustain and deepen involvement of those contributing and critical to the response such as PLWHA organizations
- Move beyond the organizations already involved and reach out to optimally engage a broad range of sectors/ actors.

**From Policy to Action:** In engaging non-state entities in an expanded response to the epidemic, the UNAIDS Secretariat:

- Fosters and supports global, regional and country level partnerships which include linkages between and among civil society, private sector, philanthropy, media, and with particular attention to organizations of people living with HIV/AIDS
- Supports governments and UN agencies in developing partnerships with non-state entities. This includes support for approaches intended to increase participation, improve connectedness of efforts and strengthen the various participants' capacity for action.

## Donors

As the main advocate for global action on HIV/AIDS, UNAIDS leads, strengthens and supports an expanded response aimed at preventing the transmission of HIV, providing care and support, reducing the vulnerability of individuals and communities to HIV/AIDS, and alleviating the impact of the epidemic. To fulfil this mandate, UNAIDS is supported by voluntary contributions from governments, foundations, corporations, private groups (for example, students, universities, sporting clubs, etc.) and individuals.

In 2003, more than US$118.5 million was received from 30 governments, philanthropic organizations, individuals from around the world and others. The largest donors were the Netherlands followed by Norway, the United States, Sweden, the United Kingdom and Japan. In 2004, 35 governments contributed to UNAIDS.

## PRESIDENT'S EMERGENCY PLAN FOR AIDS RELIEF

The President's Emergency Plan For AIDS Relief (PEPFAR/ Emergency Plan) is President Bush's pledge of $15 billion over five years (2003-2008) to fight the HIV/AIDS pandemic. As the largest international health initiative ever initiated by one nation to address a single disease, the program hopes to provide antiretroviral treatment (ART) to 2 million HIV-infected people in resource-limited settings, to prevent 7 million new infections, and to support care for 10 million people (the "2-7-10 goals").

The U.S. Leadership Against HIV/AIDS, Tuberculosis, and Malaria Act of 2003 (or the Global AIDS Act) established the State Department Office of the Global AIDS Coordinator to oversee all international AIDS funding and programming. Ambassador Mark R. Dybul has been the U.S. Global AIDS Coordinator since July 2006.

### Focus Countries

PEPFAR prioritizes resource-limited countries with high HIV/AIDS prevalence rates. The 15 current "focus countries" include Botswana, Cote d'Ivoire, Ethiopia, Guyana, Haiti, Kenya, Mozambique, Namibia, Nigeria, Rwanda, South Africa, Tanzania, Uganda, Vietnam, and Zambia. While most of the $15 billion for this program will be spent on these focus countries, $4 billion is allocated for programs elsewhere, and for HIV/ AIDS research.

### Prevention

To slow the spread of the epidemic, PEPFAR supports a variety of prevention programs: the ABC approach (Abstain, Be faithful, and correct and consistent use of Condoms); prevention of mother to child transmission (PMTCT) interventions; and programs focusing on blood safety, injection safety, secondary prevention ("prevention with positives"), counseling and education.

### Treatment

In addition to providing antiretroviral therapy (ART), PEPFAR supports prevention and treatment of opportunistic infections, as well as services to prevent and treat malaria, tuberculosis, waterborne illness, and other acute infections. PEPFAR supports training and salaries for personnel (including clinicians, laboratorians, pharmacists, counselors, medical records staff, outreach workers, peer educators, etc), renovation and refurbishment of health care facilities, updated laboratory equipment and distribution systems, logistics and management for drugs and other commodities. This is intended to ensure the sustainability of PEPFAR services in host countries, enabling long-term management of HIV/AIDS.

### Care

For those who have already been infected with HIV/AIDS, PEPFAR provides HIV counseling, resources for maintaining financial stability, etc. Special care is given to orphans and vulnerable children (OVCs) and services are provided that meet the unique needs of women and girls, including victims of sex trafficking, rape, abuse, and exploitation. Finally, the Emergency Plan works closely with country leaders, military groups, faith-based organizations, etc. in an attempt to eliminate stigma.

## PROGRAMS

PEPFAR establishes bilateral programs in host countries and also works closely with multilateral partners, such as the Global Fund to Fight AIDS, Tuberculosis and Malaria and the World Health Organization (WHO), as well as local Faith-Based Organizations. PEPFAR also endorses the international principles of the "Three Ones":-one national plan, one national coordinating authority, and one national monitoring and evaluation system in each of the host countries in which organizations work.

## ACCOUNTABILITY

PEPFAR reports to Congress on an annual basis, providing programmatic and financial data as required by law. The Second Annual Report to Congress on the President's Emergency Plan for AIDS Relief is available on the official PEPFAR website, as are more specific reports, financial information and other information.

PEPFAR is exempt from the Mexico City Policy, also known as the "global gag rule."

## CRITICISM

Public health experts and non-profit organizations have questioned the tactics and effectiveness of PEPFAR programs, including requirements mandating that one-third of prevention spending be directed towards abstinence-only programs.

According to its critics, PEPFAR is influenced too heavily by American political and social groups with "moral" rather than public health agendas. PEPFAR Watch, a website run by the Center for Health and Gender Equity and Health GAP, notes that the legislation behind PEPFAR "contains several restrictions, including those on funding for prevention activities and on organizations working with commercial sex workers." PEPFAR has also refused to fund effective yet "taboo" safe needle exchange programs to prevent HIV transmission among drug users.

An early criticism was that PEPFAR initially supported only branded antiretroviral drugs instead of cheaper generic versions; this has become less of an issue since distribution of generic drugs began in late 2005.

As above, the accuracy of PEPFAR reporting has also been questioned, and internal audits have identified areas where improvement in monitoring and evaluation-particularly of prevention services-is needed.

## NAMES PROJECT AIDS MEMORIAL QUILT

### The AIDS Quilt

The AIDS Memorial Quilt is an enormous quilt made as a memorial to and celebration of the lives of people who have died of AIDS-related causes.

The Quilt is maintained and displayed by The NAMES Project Foundation and was started in 1987 in San Francisco by Cleve Jones and a group of volunteers. At the time of its creation, most people who died of AIDS-related causes did not receive funerals and their remains were in fact refused by many funeral homes and cemeteries. Lacking a memorial service or grave site, The Quilt was often the only opportunity survivors had to remember and celebrate their loved ones' lives. The Quilt was last displayed in full on The Mall in Washington, D.C., in 1996.

Typically very personalized, individual quilt panels are created by the loved ones of someone who has died of AIDS-related causes. Each 3' by 6' panel is the size of a human grave and the panels are donated to The NAMES Project Foundation where they are grouped with other similar panels and assembled into 12' by 12' sections, called "blocks". These blocks are what are seen at local displays of The Quilt, and typically contain 8 individual panels.

The creation of a panel can be very emotional as memorable photos, favorite sayings, or favorite pieces of clothing of the deceased are attached to the panel. Displays of The Quilt can be somber experiences as people view the panels, make connections with those memorialized and realize the tragic loss of life.

In observance of National HIV-Testing Day in June 2004 the 1,000 newest blocks were displayed by the Foundation on the Ellipse in Washington, D.C. This was the largest display of The Quilt since it was last displayed in its entirety in October 1996. In fact, the 1,000 blocks displayed consisted of every panel submitted at or after the 1996 display.

Techniques used included patchwork, applique, embroidery, fabric painting, collage, spray paint and needlepoint.

Items and materials included in the panels:

- Fabrics, e.g. lace, suede, leather, mink, taffeta, also Bubble wrap and other kinds of plastic and even metal.
- Decorative items like pearls, quartz crystals, rhinestones, sequins, feathers, buttons.
- Clothing, e.g. jeans, T-shirts, gloves, boots, hats, uniforms, jackets, flip-flops.
- Items of a personal nature, such as human hair, cremation ashes, wedding rings, merit badges and other awards, car keys.

- Unusual items, e.g. stuffed animals, records, jockstraps, condoms and a bowling ball.

The NAMES Project Foundation is now headquartered in Atlanta, Georgia, but has 21 chapters in the United States and more than 40 affiliate organisations world-wide. The AIDS Memorial Quilt itself is also housed in Atlanta when not being displayed, and continues to grow, currently consisting of 5,748 blocks (more than 44,000 individual memorial panels).

The NAMES Project was nominated for a Nobel Peace Prize in 1989.

On December 1, 2006, a "Digital Quilt", commemorating the original AIDS Memorial Quilt, was unveiled as part of Project Stitch, a youth-targeted initiative organised by AIDS Vancouver, an AIDS service organisation based in Vancouver, Canada, along with other community partners. Project Stitch and the Digital Quilt are a continuing initiative, with submissions to the quilt being made online and at educational workshops for youth.

# 8

# Women of India Effected from HIV/AIDS

At the Vasavya Mahila Mandali home for vulnerable women and children in the city of Vijayavada in the southern Indian state of Andhra Pradesh, 23-year-old Nagmani clutches her five-year-old daughter in her lap.

Neither smiles. The doctors say both of them are traumatised. In January Nagmani's husband died of Aids.

"After my husband died my parents in-law threw me out of their house," she says.

"My brother's wife didn't want me in my family's house either. I had no place to go, that's why my daughter and I came here."

Test results show Nagmani too is HIV-positive, but that's too much for her to cope with. She refuses to accept she is infected.

India already has over five million HIV-positive people.

Global progress towards the UN Millennium Development Goal of halting and reversing the spread of Aids by 2015 is minimal, and India is likely to find it particularly hard to fulfil.

Currently 39% of HIV-positive Indians are women.

The government here says it is trying to promote awareness.

But health workers fear unless there is a massive campaign to combat the widespread ignorance of HIV, especially among women, the situation will soon get much worse.

"Not only the illiterate women, but the so-called educated women also are not aware of HIV/Aids.

"That is the pity of the situation among women here," says Dr Deeksha, the medical director of Vasavya Mahila Mandali, which-in addition to running the home for vulnerable women-also works in HIV awareness and cares for women in Andhra Pradesh.

### Taboos

Sex is still largely a taboo subject in India, which makes education even more difficult, according to Dr Anbumani Ramadoss, the Indian health minister.

"We are trying to sensitise the husband in the first phase, saying don't do this and don't do that and try to be faithful and abstinent.

"It's a closely-knit community out there, and getting into the community, it takes a lot of work and energy," he says.

But the Indian government has come under fire from Aids activists, who accuse it of not doing enough to promote awareness or care.

"I think it's pretty much out of hand as far as I'm concerned," says Anjali Gopalan of the Naz Foundation.

"We're seeing a tremendous rise in numbers of people who are living with HIV," she says.

"We are seeing a rise in the number of orphans, so I think the window for opportunity that we did have even five years ago is not there any more."

### High-risk Groups

Government prevention programmes have focused until very recently almost exclusively on high-risk groups such as sex workers, gay men and lorry drivers.

Consequently it is still largely seen as a disease confined to these groups by those Indians who are aware of HIV.

Accurate figures on HIV awareness are not available, but Dr Deeksha of Vasavya Mahila Mandali estimates at least 70%

of women in the rural areas where she works have not heard of the virus.

The first time Lakshmi, 33, who lives in a slum just outside Vijayavada, learnt of HIV was when she received her positive test results.

"My husband is a truck driver and I got HIV through him. I had never heard of HIV or condoms before that and because I can't read, I couldn't understand any of the posters or banners."

Lakshmi's 12-year-old son died of Aids two years ago, which was when both she and her husband discovered they too were HIV-positive.

"I was very much afraid about my HIV status because no one wanted to touch us and people wouldn't let us into their houses.

"There's so much stigma," she says. "As a woman, I didn't want to go outside.

"Then I found a doctor who would touch me and he told me it's nothing to worry about and then I got the willpower to live."

Lakshmi has begun her own fight against ignorance by educating and counselling women in her area about HIV.

But it is only through people like her and the work of a handful of non-governmental organisations that HIV awareness is being spread amongst women in rural India.

According to Anjali Gopalan, the lack of services and awareness programmes is at a critical stage.

"We haven't really improved the services that exist at ground level and there seems to be such a tremendous resistance even now," she says. Without a massive increase in awareness programmes-particularly aimed at women-India risks an epidemic which could cost millions of lives.

## "WITHOUT MY CONSENT"-WOMEN AND HIV-RELATED STIGMA IN INDIA

"I used to watch a serial on TV about AIDS. The woman got it from her husband, and when he died they [in-laws] threw her out of the house. This happens in real life." "Men don't carry condoms in their pockets. And even if he has one, he won't use it... When he wants to do it, he just tells me to come aside."

(March 2003) Both are voices of women in Delhi, but they could be from anywhere in this country of 1 billion people. For millions of Indian women, sexual intercourse is not a question of choice but rather one of survival and duty. Married before she has grown beyond adolescence, her fertility and her relationship to her husband are often the source of an Indian woman's social identity, notes the study Living Under a Shadow: Gender and HIV/AIDS in Delhi.

### Focus on Social Inequalities is Key

Sonam Rana, regional program coordinator of the United Nations Development Programme's HIV and Development Programme, sees the HIV/AIDS epidemic in India as inextricably tied to the social and cultural values and economic relationships between men and women and within communities. While social inequalities facilitate its spread in the country, the virus, in turn, reflects and reinforces these inequalities. Women are the least powerful because Indian society praises patriarchy and male sexuality and mourns the births of daughters. (The Census of India 2001 highlighted a worsening sex ratio of 933 females to 1,000 males.) In addition, there is an absence of choice at the individual and systemic levels, whether it is the choice to use a condom or even to have sex.

In the last few years, prevention experts have shifted from looking at the HIV/AIDS epidemic solely as a health issue to focusing on other factors that increase vulnerability to infection. For women, low economic and social status, abuse and violence, as well as limited legal and social protection increase their vulnerability to HIV/AIDS.

### Awareness of HIV/AIDS Low

The National AIDS Control Organisation (NACO), which was set up in 1992 to develop a multisectoral program for HIV/AIDS prevention, estimates that nearly 4 million people were living with the virus by March 2002. But this is a silent epidemic. According to UNAIDS, 95 percent of Indians with HIV do not know they have the virus, which may also be masked by tuberculosis and other opportunistic infections. In addition, fear of hostile reactions from the community and at the workplace-in the absence of protective policies-and a general lack of knowledge drive the virus further underground.

Knowledge of HIV/AIDS continues to be surprisingly low. The National Family Health Survey, 1998-99 shows that only four out of 10 women of reproductive age have heard of AIDS. Awareness is much lower among rural and less educated women. Only 18 percent of illiterate women have heard of AIDS, compared with 92 percent of women who had at least completed high school.

Even among those who have heard about HIV/AIDS, awareness of how to prevent infection is low. Nearly all respondents in four community-based studies on gender and HIV/AIDS sponsored by the United Nations Development Fund for Women (UNIFEM) in 2000 viewed the condom primarily as a contraceptive device. Conducted in two Indian cities, Pune and Delhi, and two states, Assam and Andhra Pradesh, the study showed that the most common perceptions were "How can you tell him to use a condom if you are pregnant?" and "When I am using a contraceptive, there is no need for my husband to use anything."

## Burdens of Blame and Care Fall on Women

Most Indians refuse to believe that heterosexual transmission accounts for 80 percent of infections in India. The virus has expanded the boundaries of high-risk groups to include adolescent girls (married and single); married women of reproductive age; sexually active single women; sex workers; college and university students; pregnant women; and women survivors of sexual abuse and rape. Women constitute 25 percent of known AIDS cases in the country, according to NACO. Data indicate that seven of 10 women affected by HIV are from poor rural and poor urban communities.

Yet recent mortality and morbidity data indicate that women remain providers and not receivers of health care. Shalini Bharat of the Tata Institute of Social Sciences (TISS) in Mumbai revealed in a 2001 study that while the majority of those who shared their HIV status with their families were looked after by family members, it was largely men who received such care.

Women with HIV are subjected to various forms of violence and discrimination based on gender. They could be refused shelter, denied a share of household property, refused access to treatment and care, or blamed for a husband's HIV diagnosis.

"When my in-laws got to know about my husband's HIV status they immediately blamed me for giving him the infection," said a 23-year-old woman.

In cases where a man has admitted he had sexual relations with sex workers, the burden of blame still falls on the wife for failing to "satisfy" her husband, according to the 1996 household study, Facing the Challenge. Women with the virus may also be physically abused. Deaths due to injury and sexual violence of women with HIV are on the increase. A 1997 study by K. Sathiamoorthy and Suniti Solomon showed 48.7 percent of women living with HIV experienced violence in the home.

## BREAKING THE SILENCE

From a position of denial that HIV/AIDS could be a problem in India, Prime Minister Atal Bihari Vajpayee said in a December 1998 speech, "HIV/AIDS today is the most serious public health problem facing India." While three states-Maharashtra, Tamil Nadu, and Manipur-lead in infection rates, cases have been reported in almost every Indian state. The virus is no longer confined to urban centers but is rapidly spreading to the rural areas, moving from those practicing high-risk behavior to the general population in some regions. Various studies have found high levels of HIV/AIDS among selected groups of women who have remained monogamous in their marriages.

In Pune (Maharashtra state), one study showed that of the 400 women visiting clinics for sexually transmitted infections (STIs), 93 percent were married and 91 percent had sex with their husbands only. All had at least one STI and 13.6 percent tested positive for HIV, according to the 1999 UNAIDS report, AIDS: 5 Years Since ICPD. The prevalence pattern is shifting toward women and young people, resulting in an increase of mother-to-child transmission and pediatric HIV infection.

Women account for 25 percent of new infections, according to the UNAIDS India Annual Report 2000.

### Almost Half of Rural Indian Women Have Not Heard of HIV/AIDS, Report Says

About 46% of women living in rural areas of India have not heard of HIV/AIDS, according to a recently released report from the Indian government's National Family Health Survey, which is supported by UNICEF and the British and U.S. governments, Reuters reports. According to the report, 57% of women nationwide have heard of the disease, compared with 80% of men. The Indian government has focused its HIV/AIDS prevention efforts on high-risk groups, such as commercial sex workers and injection drug users, rather than on the general population, according to Reuters. An unnamed government official said that the government is "expanding prevention efforts among the general population in rural areas, especially women, over the next five years." Anjali Gopalan—head of the HIV/AIDS advocacy group Naz Foundation India—said the report "shows women don't have access to information, translating into more women getting infected."

According to Reuters, women account for 40% of HIV cases in the country. Many women in rural areas contract the virus from their husbands, who travel to cities and visit commercial sex workers, Reuters reports. HIV/AIDS advocates are urging the government to train health workers and send them to rural areas in an effort to educate rural women about the virus (Zaheer, Reuters, 2/23).

### Women are Increasingly Vulnerable to HIV/AIDS.

- o Nearly half of the 40 million people currently living with HIV/AIDS (PLWHA) are female, up from 41 percent in 1997 and 35 percent in 1985.
- o In every region of the world, more women are living with HIV than ever before. This number increased by 1 million between 2004 and 2006.
- o In sub-Saharan Africa, 59 percent of PLWHA are female.
- o In the Caribbean 51 percent of PLWHA are women, up from 30 percent in 1999.

- In India 39 percent of PLWHA are women.
- In China, women constituted 39 percent of reported HIV cases in 2004, up from 25 percent two years earlier.
- In the U.S., the number of women living with AIDS increased 15 percent between 1999 and 2003, compared with 1 percent in men. The rate of new HIV or AIDS diagnoses was 21 times higher among African American women than among white women in 2004 and AIDS is the leading cause of death in African American women aged 25 to 34.
- In Russia, more than 40 percent of newly reported HIV infections in 2005 were among women-a larger proportion than ever before.

Young people, especially young women, are disproportionately at risk.

- Young people (aged 15-24) accounted for 40 percent of the 4.1 million new HIV infections in 2005.
- Young women account for 62 percent of PLWHA between the ages of 15 and 24.
- In sub-Saharan Africa, 76 percent of HIV-positive young people are female.
- In South Asia, 62 percent are female. In India, the number of young women living with HIV/AIDS is twice that of young men.
- In Lesotho, for women aged 18-19 years, less than 10 percent are HIV-positive, but by the time they celebrate their 22nd birthday, 30 percent will have acquired HIV, and by the time they reach 24 years, almost 40 percent will have been infected.
- HIV prevalence among girls under 18 is four to seven times higher than among boys in many countries of eastern and southern Africa.
- In Uganda, the risk of HIV infection doubles for girls 15-19 who have male partners ten or more years older.
- Among teens 13-19 in the United States, girls account for 50 percent of new HIV infections.

Women and girls do not have access to comprehensive information and services.

- o Only 26 percent of girls 10-19 in Somalia have heard of AIDS, and only 1 percent know how to protect themselves from the virus.
- o In Bangladesh, less than 20 percent of married women have heard of AIDS.
- o In India, if AIDS education is even offered in schools, it is to young people 15 and older. Yet 42 percent of boys and 69 percent of girls 15-17 are not in school.
- o One in four young South Africans believe that sex with a virgin can cure HIV/AIDS.

The biggest HIV/AIDS risk for many women and girls is marriage.

- o More than four-fifths of new infections in women result from sex with their husband or primary partners.
- o In Ghana, married women are almost three times more likely to be HIV-infected than women who have never been married.
- o In India, 27 percent of male clients of male sex workers are married or living with a female partner.
- o Throughout countries of Africa and Latin America, more than 80 percent of adolescents who have had unprotected sex in the last week are married.

Sexual coercion and violence lead to a greater chance of infection.

- o One in three women around the world will be raped, beaten, coerced into sex, or otherwise abused in her lifetime.
- o Fearing violence or rejection, 58 percent of African girls avoid discussing condom use with their partners. Yet in couples where only one partner is infected with HIV, consistent and correct condom use provides the HIV negative person with a near zero risk of infection.
- o Women in South Africa who are in relationships with violent or domineering men are 50 percent more likely

to contract HIV than women not involved in abusive relationships.

- o A study among high school students in Swaziland found that almost one in five of the sexually active female students' first sexual experience had been coerced.
- o In South Africa, 30 percent of girls say their first intercourse was forced, and 71 percent have experienced sex against their will.

## SOCIO-ECONOMIC BACKGROUND

With more than a billion people, one of the fastest economic growth rates in the world since the 1980s and a robust Information Technology industry that is projected to earn about US $ 50 billion by 2008, India is a country of striking contrasts.

With more than a quarter of the population living below poverty line, making the numbers in absolute terms (2002) living below the poverty line, the country has the highest concentration of poverty anywhere in the world. The country accounts for 40 per cent of the world's poor and its social indicators are still poor my most measures of human development. At 6.0 per cent of GDP (March, 2004), its fiscal deficit is one of the highest in the world.

- More than half of all children under the age of four are malnourished and 30 percent of newborns are significantly underweight.
- India adds 16 million people every year to its population, just two million less than the entire population of Australia
- 60 per cent of the women are anaemic.
- Maternal deaths at 540/1000 account for almost 25 percent of the world's childbirth-related deaths.
- Almost half of Indian women are illiterate though it has the second largest education system in the world after China.
- India has the largest remaining pool of polio transmission in the world.

But the poor indicators do not articulate India's achievements.

The general condition of India's population has improved since the 1970s. Average life expectancy at birth has increased from 50 years to 63.9, the infant mortality rate has fallen by half to about 67 per 1,000 live births, and the crude birth rate has fallen to about 25 per thousand population.

India's national family welfare program has helped move the country about two-thirds of the way toward its goal of replacement-level fertility. However, population growth and the impending strain on the environment, natural resources, and social services still pose a threat to India's development.

Despite some improvement, India's women remain significantly more malnourished than men. Bias against women and girls is reflected in the demographic ratio of 933 females for every 1,000 males. The country's maternal mortality rate at 540 is very high, particularly in rural areas it is even higher.

Although declining, largely preventable diseases such as leprosy, tuberculosis, cataract blindness, and malaria continue to account for 50 percent of reported illness, and around 470 deaths per 100,000. Despite a decade of polio initiatives under India's immunisation program, India accounted for more than two-thirds of polio cases reported worldwide in 1998.

India made modest increases in primary education enrolment rates in the 1990s.

The rise in literacy rates over the last decade indicates India's progress in education. In the last decade, the overall literacy rate increased from 52 percent to 65.38 percent. Yet almost half of Indian women are still illiterate; about 40 million primary school-age children are not in school (mostly girls and those from the poorest and socially-excluded households); and only about one-third of an age group completes the constitutionally prescribed eight years of education.

## HIV SITUATION

An estimated 5.1 million Indians are currently living with HIV. Concentrated in seven states with over 1% antenatal prevalence in four of the industrialized western and southern states of India (specifically Andhra Pradesh, Karnataka, Maharashtra and Tamil Nadu) and in the north-eastern states of Manipur and Nagaland, the epidemic is highly heterogenous. Although data gathered by NACO in 2004 has revealed that HIV prevalence has stabilised in at least Tamil Nadu, Andhra Pradesh, Karnataka, and Maharashtra, it is increasing in at-risk populations in other states. As a result, overall HIV prevalence has continued to rise.

A significant proportion of new infections is occurring in women who are married and who have been infected by husbands who either currently or in the past) frequented sex workers. Commercial sex (along with injecting drug use, in the cases of Nagaland and Tamil Nadu) serves as a major driver of the epidemic in most parts of India. Surveys in 2003 found 14% of commercial sex workers in Karnataka and 19% in Andhra Pradesh were infected with HIV. In Mysore, 26% of sex workers were HIV positive, according to a 2005 survey.

**Commercial Sex and Condom Use**

Surveys carried out in various parts of India in 2001 found that 30% of street-based sex workers did not know that condoms prevented HIV infection, and in some states, such as Haryana, fewer than half of all sex workers (brothel-and street-based) knew that condoms prevented HIV. Even four years later there seemed to have been no improvement in the situation. Surveys in 2005 again revealed that 42% thought they could tell whether a client had HIV on the basis of his physical appearance. At the same time, another study in Mysore revealed that only 14% of sex workers used condoms consistently with clients and that 91% of them never used condoms during sex with their regular partners.

There are some exceptions, of course. Among them are the sex workers of Kolkata's Sonagachi red-light area (in West Bengal) who have shown that safer sex programmes that empower sex workers can curb the spread of HIV. Condom use in Sonagachi has risen as high as 85% and HIV prevalence among commercial sex workers declined to under 4% in 2004 (having exceeded 11% in 2001). In Mumbai, by contrast, available data suggest that sporadic and piecemeal efforts to promote condom use during commercial sex have not been as effective; there, HIV prevalence among female sex workers has not fallen below 52% since 2000 (NACO, 2004).

## Injecting Drug Use

In the north-east of India, HIV transmission is concentrated chiefly among drug injectors and their sexual partners (some of whom also buy or sell sex), especially in the states of Manipur, Mizoram and Nagaland, all of which lie adjacent to the drug-trafficking 'Golden Triangle' zone (Solomon et al., 2004). Some 20% of female sex workers said they injected drugs, according to behavioural surveillance. In other north-eastern states, about half as many sex workers have reported injecting drugs.

Harm reduction efforts (including needle and syringe exchange, as well as limited drug substitution programmes) were introduced in some states, such as Manipur. There, in 2003 the HIV prevalence among drug injectors was 24%-the lowest levels detected among injecting drug users in that state since 1998. Elsewhere the epidemics among drug injectors appear to be well established, with HIV prevalence having reached 14% in Nagaland in 2000-2003, for example.

But not only in the North-east, there has been a sharp rise in HIV infections among drug injectors in the southern state of Tamil Nadu, where 39% were HIV-infected in 2003, compared with 25% in 2001. In Chennai, Tamil Nadu, almost two thirds (64%) of injectors were HIV-positive, according to sentinel surveillance done in 2003.

## Other Factors

Relatively little is known about the role of sex between men in India's HIV epidemic. The few studies that have examined this complex dimension of sexuality in India have found that significant numbers of men do have sex with other men. One study, undertaken among residents slum areas in Chennai, has found that 6% of men had had sexual intercourse with another man. Almost 7% of the men who had sex with other men were HIV-positive, and more than half them were married.

Poverty combined with low status does not allow a vast majority of women to negotiate safe sex, and thus makes them vulnerable to the disease. Like in many other developing countries, migration and mobility not only makes people vulnerable to HIV but is also a contributing factor to the spread of the disease.

**Government Response**

Beginning with the establishment of a National AIDS Control Program (NACP), managed by a small unit within the Ministry of Health and Family Welfare, the government has over time scaled up its response considerably. The Government has already implemented various programmes and amended rules regarding blood safety and established a decentralized mechanism to facilitate effective state-level responses to HIV prevention programmes, through NACP I and II. It is currently preparing for NACP III. The design of NACP 3 includes a complex consultative process. State specific and nationwide consultations are being held with national stakeholders such as PLWHA networks, local and international NGOs, experts and practitioners of HIV control initiatives, as well as international development partners.

**NACP I and II**

The NACP 1 which lasted from 1992-1999 met several challenges-from limited capacity to denial and low commitment—headlong and registered some success. The achievements included capacity building in managerial and technical aspects of the programme in all states and union territories, setting up of training centres for personnel in management of HIV and strengthening some 500 STD clinics. Importantly, blood transfusion without license was made illegal and by the end of the project term in 1999, there were no unlicensed blood banks. Also, 154 zonal blood testing centres were set up and 815 public sector and voluntary blood banks strengthened. Surveillance capacity was developed in 140 centres and 180 sentinel sites nationwide.

The NACP II which finished its run in March 2006, sought to shift focus from raising awareness to changing behaviour through interventions. The Project aimed at evidence-based planning, prevention and an expanded mandate for care and support for people living with HIV/AIDS.

Priority was given to setting up annual sentinel surveillance, HIV case detection, mapping of high-risk groups and behavioural surveillance. Building on the experience of the first phase, there was a twin drive to focus on coverage amongst high risk groups like sex workers, truck drivers and injecting drug users and to make the programme multi-sectoral. It resulted in a strongly decentralized programme with the responsibility of implementation vested with the states. Flexible State AIDS Societies were formed with stronger mechanisms for state level programme management. The outcomes envisaged in the NACP II were to keep HIV seroprevalence below 5% of the adult population in high prevalence states, below 3% in the moderate prevalence states and below 1% in the low prevalence states.

**Anti-retroviral Treatment**

As Indian-manufactured generic drugs entered the market and costs of anti-retroviral treatment registered a sharp decline, conditions were feasible, to some extent, for the government to provide free anti-retroviral treatment. From April 1, 2004, anti-retroviral treatment is being provided free of cost at government hospitals in six high prevalence states of Tamil Nadu, Andhra Pradesh, Maharashtra, Karnakata, Manipur, Nagaland and Delhi.

Additionally, the government priorised three categories for initial outreach: 1) the HIV positive women who access government antinatal clinics, 2) children up to 15 years of age and 3) adults with full blown AIDS who access government hospitals for care and treatment. Between 2004-05, the government sought to increase the number of ART centres from 8 to 25.

**Research, Vaccine Trials**

Almost 60 microbicidial products or compounds are under development world-wide and some of these have entered into phase II clinical trials. In India, research and development is being undertaken on polyherbal neem based microbicide tablets.

Phase I trial of this microbicide was conducted by National Institute of Research on Reproductive Health, Mumbai and PGI, Chandigarh. The product has been found safe. Extended and initial efficacy trials are being conducted by National AIDS Research Institute, Pune.

Condom use, mutual monogamy and abstinence are not any real options for a lot of women, specially in a developing country where poverty and gender inequality is high. For those who lack the power of negotiating sex safe, microbicides are a potentially lifesaving alternative to condoms.

As regards vaccines, several of these have been reviewed to select the most appropriate one for India. A multistakeholder Advisory Board is in place to deliberate the legal, ethical and socio-behavioural issues related to vaccine trials in the country. In July 2005, India and America agreed to speed up the review of generic antiretroviral drugs by the U.S. Food and Drug Administration. (eight of the 10 drugs approved so far are made in India.)

## Corporate Support and HIV/AIDS

By corporate sector's own admission, their proactive engagement into HIV/AIDS in India has till recently remained piecemeal. From late 2005, however, there has been a flurry of activity with business houses coming together to chalk out a roadmap in establishing corporate HIV/AIDS programs targeted at the workforce and/or community of private sector companies. A mid-2005 Global Health Initiative study of the World Economic Forum had revealed that just 7% of Indian companies expected HIV/AIDS to have any serious impact on their operations. The report "Business & HIV/AIDS: A Healthier Partnership?" surveyed 11,000 business leaders in 117 countries between January and May 2005. Of the Indian corporate bodies surveyed, only 11% had any written policy to combat discrimination in promotion, pay or benefits based on HIV status. About 31% reported having an informal policy, while 52% had no policy to face the expected challenge.

The report observes that 76% of Indian companies surveyed claim to have a prevention programme, while only 29% have provision for any voluntary testing against the global average of 33%. In 50% of cases there was no provision for voluntary testing, 45% had no facilities to distribute condoms, and 67% had no treatment programme.

On the positive side, 14% had an active policy to protect workers, with 10% ensuring access to anti-retroviral treatment, 19% to promotion of condom usage, and 29% to providing voluntary testing facilities.

In September 2005 CoRE-BCSD India-a 52 company strong platform for Indian corporates to accomplish their mission for sustainable development-initiated action to strengthen Indian industry's response to the HIV epidemic. The process is expected to generate a dialogue in the company on a disease that concerns everyone. Three possible areas where business houses could initiate, support/scale up awareness and prevent the spread of the epidemic were identified:

- their workplace-by raising awareness about HIV/AIDS and promoting prevention among employees in the workplace, and by extending such education programs throughout their operations and to partners in their supply chain;
- their clinical facilities-by training medical and clinical staff on HIV/AIDS and sexually transmitted infections (STIs), i.e. modes of transmission, prevention (with a special focus on universal precautions related to HIV infection in clinical settings), basic counseling skills, syndromic management of STIs, opportunistic infections related to HIV and anti-retroviral treatment therapies;
- their communities-by supporting or scaling-up the awareness and prevention efforts within high risk or vulnerable populations around their operations, particularly the migrant workers and trucking community which some companies see as key stakeholders, or with whom they interact on a day-to-day basis.

Intervention also includes forming an action plan that will be reviewed on a regular basis and drafting a HIV/AIDS policy that will be promoted at all levels at the workplace.

In March 2006, Global Business Coalition on HIV/AIDS (GBC) and the Confederation of Indian Industry (CII) jointly initiated a project engaging corporations involved in Business Process Outsourcing. GBC's work with India's growing BPO industry is supported by Prime Minister Manmohan Singh and GBC Corporate Advisory Board member Ratan N. Tata.

### Donors

India receives technical assistance and funding from a variety of UN partners and bilateral donors. Bilateral donors such as USAID, CIDA, and DFID have been involved since the early 1990s at the state level in a number of states. USAID has committed more than US$70 million since 1992, CIDA US$11 million, and DFID close to US$200 million.

The number of major financers and the amount of funding available has increased significantly in the last year. Since 2004, the Gates Foundation has pledged US$200 million for the next five years, the Global Fund has approved US$54 million for HIV/AIDS for projects in rounds two, three and four. DFID has also increased its financing and is considering the inclusion of additional states. Other more recent donors include DANIDA, SIDA, the Clinton Foundation and the European Union.

## HIV/AIDS ESTIMATES

### HIV in India-A fast spreading epidemic

**1986:** First case of HIV detected in Chennai.

**1990:** HIV levels among High Risk Groups like Sex workers and STD clinic attendants in Maharashtra and amongst Injecting Drug Users in Manipur reaches over 5 percent.

**1994:** HIV no longer restricted to high risk groups in Maharashtra, but spreading into the general population. HIV also spreading to the states of Gujarat and Tamil Nadu where high risk groups have over 5 percent HIV prevalence.

**1998:** Rapid HIV spread in the four large southern states, not only in high-risk groups but also in the general population where it has reached over 1 percent. Infection rate among antenatal women reaches 3.3 in Namakkal in Tamil Nadu and 5.3 in Churachandpur in Manipur. Among IDUs in

Churachandpur it crosses 76 percent and in Mumbai, 64.4 per cent.

**1999:** The infection rate in antenatal women in Namakkal rises to 6.5. About 60 per cent of the sex workers in some Mumbai sites are infected. Infection rates among STD patients have reached up to 30 percent in Andhra Pradesh and 14-60 per cent in Maharashtra. About 64.4 percent IDUs at one of the sites in Mumbai and 68.4 percent in Chruachandpur are infected.

**2001:** Infection crosses one per cent in six states. These states account for 75 per cent of the country's estimated HIV cases. The Prime Minister addresses the Chief Ministers of high prevalence states and urges them to intensify prevention activities.

**2002:** In year 2003 there has been an increase of about 6 lakh infections (4.58 million). This increase has been noticed primarily in states of Karnataka, Rajasthan, West Bengal, Tamil Nadu, Gujarat, Bihar, Madhya Pradesh and Rajasthan. There is no significant increase in HIV infections in the country. India continues to be in the category of low prevalence countries with overall prevalence of less than 1 percent.

## AN OVERVIEW OF THE SPREAD AND PREVALENCE OF HIV/AIDS IN INDIA

### National HIV Policy India

- Ministry of Human Resource Development (Dept. of Youth & Sports) involved in implementation of "Universities Talk AIDS" Programme of the National Service Scheme covering 158 universities, 5000 colleges and 2000 senior secondary schools.
- National Council of Education Research & Training (NCERT) involved in development of school curriculum package for integration of HIV/AIDS into school education (extra-curricular activities).
- A national consultation on the integration of HIV/AIDS into school education has been organised under the auspices of UNAIDS by UNESCO, UNFPA, and UNICEF with financial support from NACO and the active

involvement of the Department of Education and five key states where these activities have been implemented. Follow-up is expected between NACO and the Department of Education with support from the UN System.

- Nehru Yuvak Kendra (NYK) involved in the implementation of non-formal educational approaches and rural outreach programmes on HIV/AIDS through its national volunteer network in communities in the country.
- Ministry of Defence (Health Services) conducts IEC programmes and HIV screening within defence populations with assistance from NACO.

## World Bank Support

The Bank has provided two IDA credits to support India's National AIDS Control Program in collaboration with the World Health Organization, other donors and UNAIDS. Through its general health projects and dialogue with other South Asian countries, the Bank is focusing on HIV/AIDS as a major public health and development issue. In India, the Bank is supporting the country's ongoing program to reduce the growth of HIV infection and strengthen capacity to respond to the epidemic through information awareness efforts, focused interventions promoting behaviour change, voluntary testing and counselling, and reducing transmission by blood transfusions and occupational exposure.

## Support by Industry

Industrial federations (West Bengal Chamber of Commerce & Industry, Confederation of Indian Industry, Federation of Indian Chambers of Commerce & Industry) becoming involved in stimulating discussions on needs for industrial sectors response to HIV/AIDS. "AIDS & the Workplace" advocacy & IEC package developed by Confederation of Indian Industry (CII) with assistance from WHO/UNAIDS/USAID for promotion of industry action on HIV/AIDS prevention and workplace policies. The Trucking Corporation of India (TCI) is actively participating in a national network of NGO service providers being coordinated with support from ODA for the assurance of HIV/STD interventions for truck drivers.

**Legislation and Policies**

- Goa Public Health Act Amendment of 1985 (Section 53.I.vii) allowed the public health authorities and police discretion to isolate people with HIV/AIDS; repealed in 1996.
- Railway Board Administrative Notification of 1989 designating HIV/AIDS as "infectious disease" which can allow denial of passage; rescinded in 1996.
- Draft legislation in 1989 Session of National Parliament, which was evaluated as extremely prejudicial to rights of PLWH/As withdrawn after intervention of WHO and national authorities.
- 1992 Administrative Notification from Minister of Health & Family Welfare (GOI) to all State Governments directing them to ensure non-discriminatory access to treatment and care for PLWH/As in all Central and State Government health care institutions.
- The Government has, by Administrative Order, required the screening for HIV of all units of blood to be used for transfusion purposes.
- May 1997 Mumbai High Court Judgment held that employers cannot base employment decisions on HIV status of employee.

**HIV/AIDS**

CDC surveillance information has indicated that HIV/AIDS is a increasingly growing problem for the American Indian and Alaska Natives population. In 2004, in the 33 states with a long-term, confidential name-based HIV reporting, women accounted for 29% of the HIV/AIDS diagnoses reported for that year. An estimated 1,506 AI/AN were living with AIDS. The approximate rate of AIDS diagnosis for AI/AN adults and teens was 9.9 per 100,000 persons, the 3rd highest rate after those for African American and Hispanic adults and teens. The estimated AIDS diagnosis for their white counterparts was 7.1 per 100,000. The National Indian Women's Health Resource Center administers the HIV/AIDS Health Promotion and Education Cooperation Agreement Project which is funded by the Office of Minority Health. The goal of this project is to raise awareness and educate American Indian families of the risk factors associated and contributing to the contraction of the HIV/AIDS disease by providing culturally appropriate health education materials and trainings on how to reduce an individual and communities risk of becoming infected.

A "Train the Trainer" curriculum, which is culturally appropriate; and sensitive training materials are being developed through this project for training HIV/AIDS prevention specialists in tribal communities throughout the United States, particularly where there is a high incidence of HIV/AIDS among American Indian and Alaska Natives.

NIWHRC has also assisted with the formation of three HIV/AIDS coalitions: HEART in northeast Oklahoma, PANI HOPE in central Oklahoma, and ONNUAA in southwest Oklahoma.

HIV is a non-discriminate disease. It knows no age, sex, race, or nationality. American Indians must be educated and aware of this deadly disease.

## INDIAN WOMEN STRUGGLING WITH HIV/AIDS AND DISCLOSURE

December 2, 2003-(IRIN) Stigma and gender inequality are helping to drive HIV/AIDS in South Africa's traditionally conservative Indian communities.

Thirty-year-old Poppy Naicker is illiterate and barely able to make ends meet. But poverty and her inability to write her own name are the least of her concerns.

She is HIV-positive and has been laid low by opportunistic infections, but is shunned by the Indian community of Chatsworth near the port city of Durban, where she lives with her older sister and three teenage children in a small overcrowded council flat.

One of just a handful of Indian women in the community willing to disclose their HIV-positive status, Poppy told PlusNews she had contracted HIV from a number of encounters with men who paid her for sex that was often unprotected.

"It is difficult to refuse something if you are not sure of how good or bad it really is. Now I know about the importance of condoms and how to use them, but it is too late for me. If I knew then what I know now, I would definitely have refused unprotected sex."

Since her disclosure, her family has turned their backs on her and blame her illness on "conduct unbecoming to an Indian woman".

"Indian families always have a strong support for struggling members, but more needs to be done about educating the families about HIV/AIDS and making them speak more freely about the dangers of having the virus, and how to avoid infection," Poppy explained.

Savy Subramany, chief coordinator for the Chatsworth Community Care Centre, one of the few AIDS NGOs operating there, said the stigma against HIV/AIDS-that infection stemmed mainly from promiscuous sexual behaviour-had stopped many people in the Indian community from acknowledging their status.

Subramany said because a woman's morals and faithfulness were questioned when she tried to negotiate safer sex, couples were still engaging in unprotected sex, even when they suspected that one or both of them might be HIV-positive.

"I have come across people who suffer silently without disclosing their status, and without counselling or the appropriate care. Those who are not willing to disclose often die slowly, alone and in agony," Subramany commented.

Gender-based inequality leaves all women-not just those from the Indian community-more vulnerable to contracting HIV/AIDS because they are less able to control how, when and where sex takes place.

Forty-five-year-old Nimmi Ramsarran found herself in this situation when her husband, who often travelled for his work, suddenly became quite ill.

Nimmi said she suspected her husband might have contracted HIV during his road trips, but was afraid to confront him about it-not out of fear of her husband, whom she said she loved dearly, but rather out of her commitment to him as a traditional Indian wife.

The couple continued to engage in unprotected sexual intercourse and it was only when Nimmi's husband became worryingly ill that he decided to get a full medical examination, including an HIV test.

Following her husband's HIV-positive result, the private clinic where the tests were done advised Nimmi to be tested as well, but her result was negative.

"It was only when I was referred to the Chatsworth Community Care Centre for counselling that I met Savy, who spent many hours offering me the support and education I needed to make it through to a second HIV test," she explained.

The period between tests was gruelling for Nimmi-apart from the fear of discrimination, she also had to conceal the cause of her husband's death when he died.

"With help from the centre I was able to hold on until the second HIV test, which also turned out negative, and I have only recently overcome the fear of community members discovering mine and my dead husband's secret."

Although she is a lot more confident that her third HIV test will also turn out negative, she speaks anxiously about the episode and still refers to HIV/AIDS as "that thing".

The project manager for the University of Natal's Health Economics and AIDS Research Division, Marlene Abrahams, says more needs to be done to encourage people to speak openly about HIV/AIDS, and agrees that research on individual households could also help to bring about a greater understanding of the impact of HIV/AIDS on various cultural groups.

A recent study commissioned by former president Nelson Mandela through the Human Sciences Research Council, claims to provide the most systematic and comprehensive view available on how HIV/AIDS is affecting South Africans according to race, gender, age and geographical location. According to these findings, Indians make up 2.6 percent of the 46 million South African population, but represent 1.6 percent of all HIV-positive people. Abrahams stressed: "I feel more could done in the way of advertising campaigns, as the HIV/AIDS pandemic is also still largely regarded as a white or black person's illness and recent advertising campaigns don't do much to change that perception. It is difficult for someone of Indian... [heritage] to relate to the urgency of AIDS awareness and behavioural change when you look at a billboard and see black or white or mixed race, but no Indians."

## EMPOWERING WOMEN TO PROTECT THEMSELVES FROM HIV

On March 8, 2007, International Women's Day, Dr. Zeda F. Rosenberg, CEO, International Partnership for Microbicides said, " Recent months have brought much news, both good and bad, about new technologies currently being researched for the prevention of HIV. We have seen new data indicating that male circumcision can significantly reduce men's risk of infection, and the launch of the first vaccine efficacy trial in Africa. These are hopeful developments.

More sobering, however, was the news that trials of a microbicide candidate closed early due to concerns that the product may have increased women's risk of HIV infection. And this week, researchers announced that despite the benefits of circumcision for men, the procedure does not seem to protect the female partners of HIV-infected men who have been circumcised, at least in the short term.When all of this news is put together, sadly, women remain, for the most part, without any real protection from this disease.

We know that the current "ABC" approach (Abstaining from sex, Being faithful to one partner and using Condoms) is not enough to protect many women. Abstinence is not a realistic option for many adults, particularly those who are married or in long-term relationships. A woman may not be able to convince her partner to use condoms-or she and her partner may want to have children, which they cannot do while abstaining or using condoms. And remaining faithful to her husband cannot protect a woman whose husband is not monogamous.

Women desperately need prevention options in addition to ABC. We are obligated to provide women with better tools to keep themselves from harm. Scientific innovation can be difficult and unpredictable, and we must constantly keep in mind that the vast majority of interventions that begin the development process will fail. But when success finally occurs, millions benefit.

Developing a safe and effective microbicide that women could use to prevent HIV infection would mark a major milestone in our response to the AIDS epidemic ... All of us who are involved in HIV prevention-from laboratory scientists to ministries of health, from international donors to community health educators, and, most importantly, the tens of thousands of women and men who are volunteering to participate in clinical trials-must redouble our efforts to ensure that women, in particular, have a range of safe, effective, accessible and user-friendly tools to protect themselves from this devastating disease. We must continue to expand the microbicide pipeline with the most effective drugs and determine their safety and effectiveness in women as rapidly as possible.

Taking the next step toward combating AIDS means acting on the knowledge that what's good for the world's most vulnerable women is, in fact, good for us all."

## COMMON SEXUAL PRACTICES OF INDIAN WOMEN IN HIV/AIDS ERA-STUDY FROM CENTRAL INDIA

**Description:** 60 HIV Positive wives of Truck drivers were interviewed. All of them were aware of their husbands having sexual contacts enroute. Most of them were observant about falling health of their husbands in last 1-2 years but were not able to ask about HIV testing.

All of them came to know about HIV/AIDS only after severe infection or candidiasis or Tuberculosis. None of their husbands had been tested voluntarily before. Only one woman had suggested her husband for HIV testing. In past average sexual contacts were 5-8 per month. Their was marked reduced sexual contacts after the diagnosis. Surprisingly more than 75% women agreed that their partners had tried Anal Intercourse in their active sex life. Only two were practicing even before falling sick. Only one woman had knowledge about her husband being active member of a Gay Club of Indore.

**Issues:** Low risk spouses are getting infection in India. Sex education of average women in country is inadequate to prevent acquisition of HIV.

**Recommendation:** Sex education and awareness of HIV is still at a primitive level in average Indian society all attempts must be made to make women more aware of safe sexual practices and prevention of HIV.

Issues India is having one of the largest population of HIV/AIDS patients. With more than 40 million patients, most of the cases are acquiring HIV through sexual route. A large number of these male patients are Truck Drivers who stay away from home for long periods. A study has been done to interview the low risk spouses of these patients for their HIV status and sexual practices in past and present. This is from Indore, a city with 3 million population.

## THE FASTEST GROWING SEGMENT OF DEADLY AIDS EPIDEMIC IN INDIA

**Bangalore:** In the weeks following her husband's death from AIDS-related illnesses, Shreemathi, then 21, who became HIV positive through contact with him, tried killing herself three times, first by jumping into a well in her village in southern India, and the second time by ingesting rat poison. In her third attempt, she tried jumping off a moving train. All three times fate intervened.

What pushed her over the edge, she told India-West, was that her in-laws constantly told her that she had brought misfortune upon their family, and that she was responsible for her husband's untimely death.

They forced her to wear a white sari, symbolizing her widowhood. Implicit in that sartorial demand was a warning to put aside forever any dreams she might have harbored of carving out a new life for herself. And worst of all, they made it quite clear that she was no longer welcome in their home.

"In India, men with HIV get thrown out of their jobs; women with HIV get thrown out of their homes" and become India's invisible women, said Priti Radhakrishnan of the Bangalore chapter of the non-governmental organization,

Lawyers' Collective HIV/AIDS Unit, which promotes the fundamental rights of people living with the disease.

At the time, "my self-esteem was so low," recalled Shreemathi, now 26, the picture of confidence in her smart Punjabi suit, and a counselor at Freedom Foundation, an NGO in Bangalore's Hennur village that focuses on substance abuse and HIV/AIDS. "I saw no point in living. I wanted to end it all."

Shreemati did not want her real name to be used for fear of stigmatizing her family, and jeopardizing the marital status of her two siblings at home.

The young woman, like thousands of HIV widows in India, teetered on the brink of depression and destitution. But unlike many, she had a bachelor's degree and a few years of work experience to rely upon, first as a schoolteacher, then as an accountant.

Started in 1995, the Freedom Foundation is India's first community-based care support for those with HIV. Since its inception, it has counseled hundreds of women like Shreemathi, providing some with vocational training and turning their lives around. Aside from its Bangalore center, Freedom Foundation has chapters in other parts of Karnataka, and in Goa and Tamil Nadu. The Bangalore center also runs an AIDS orphanage. The programs are funded through international agencies, the central government and a few corporations, said Dr. Nirmala Skill, the doctor-in-charge at the Hennur village center.

Shreemathi told India-West that despite all the emotional pain she was put through by her in-laws, she does not want them to find out that their son's promiscuous behavior prior to his marriage was what led to his death. As he lay dying, he told his parents he had fallen and damaged his brain, and that doctors had told him there was nothing they could do to save his life.

"He told me he had been visiting sex workers since he was 15 years old," Shreemathi said. "But he did not want his parents to ever know that."

The young widow is among an estimated 2.4 million women in India who are known to be HIV positive. The majority of them, around 80 percent, contracted the disease from their husbands, a situation similar to South Africa. What frequently kills young women in both countries is not promiscuity, but marriage, U.N. Secretary General Kofi Annan observed.

Shreemathi said that when she first heard about her husband's HIV status, her initial reaction was anger, but it gave way to sadness after he expressed remorse for what he had done to her, she said.

"I told him that whatever has happened was my fate, so I will accept it," Shreemathi said in an interview she shoehorned between counseling sessions at the Hennur center.

AIDS workers say her fatalistic attitude is typical of most Indian women who contract the disease from their husbands.

"They've been raised to be care-givers, that's the cultural set-up," Skill said. "That's why they are sad over their husbands' condition, rarely angry."

In India, as in South Africa, AIDS is fast getting a woman's face. As Dr. S.Y. Quraishi, chief of the Indian government's 14-year-old National Aids Control Organization, observed recently, "We fear the feminization will increase in the next five years, and 50 percent of all infections will be among women."

That rate is currently a little over 40 percent, which doesn't include many women who are HIV positive but don't know it. Fears of abandonment and stigmatization keep many from getting their blood tested.

Although it's been nearly 20 years since the first AIDS cases were diagnosed in India, it's only in recent years that the magnitude of the problem has been acknowledged. The government was mostly preoccupied with making India a powerful economic growth engine so the AIDS calamity, largely looked upon as a comeuppance for promiscuous behavior, was on few radar screens.

Dr. Peter Piot, head of the UN campaign to combat AIDS, observed that a "lethal mix of apathy and denial" fuels spread of the disease.

Kapil Sibal, minister of state for Science and Technology and Ocean Development, called AIDS "a very, very lethal weapon of mass destruction," and warned that complacency has no place in the fight against AIDS because "none of us is immune to the impact of this disease."

Yet, to the majority of Indians, it is a disease that only affects someone else. At an AAPIO-sponsored talk in Milpitas, Calif., three months ago, visiting Health Minister Anbumani Ramadoss spoke of the many strides India was making on the health front under the Manmohan Singh administration. The maternity mortality rate, infant mortality rate, population explosion, stem cell research and the AIDS epidemic were some of the topics he touched upon. Then, he opened the floor up to questions from the audience. Sadly, not one person asked about the burgeoning AIDS problem in India.

## MOST INDIAN WOMEN NOT AWARE OF AIDS

More than 40 percent of women in India have not heard of AIDS. India has 5.7 million people living with HIV/AIDS, according to the United Nations, which is the world's highest case-load. But the prevalence, in the country of 1.1 billion people, is much lower than in most of Africa. According to The National Family Health Survey (NFHS), the most extensive study on health and nutrition in India, only 57 percent of women have heard of AIDS. In rural areas, where most Indians live, less than half the women-46 percent-are aware of the disease. Poor awareness among women may be fuelling the epidemic. Women don't have access to information, translating into more women getting infected. In the past few years, there has been a growing feminisation of the epidemic in India with nearly 40 percent of all those infected now being women, including housewives. Biologically, women are more susceptible to HIV, according to Action Aid-India. The lack of awareness adds to the HIV threat they face. One reason for low awareness is that the government has focused prevention efforts on high-risk groups like prostitutes and intravenous drug users, rather than on the general population. Efforts need to be expanded among the general population in rural areas, especially women, over the next five years. Many rural women have been infected by their husbands who work in the cities and visit prostitutes. Social stigma stops infected husbands from telling their wives they are HIV-positive. Many women in villages do not have television in their homes and miss out on anti-AIDS advertisements, calling for a broad-based effort to educate and empower women. Even if they do have TVs, there is no electricity in many areas. This is one way how fighting HIV is linked to the issue of general development. Activists want the government to spend more on training and sending grassroots health workers to spread AIDS education among women, especially in poor and highly populated states.

## HIV AND YOUNG AMERICAN INDIAN/ALASKA NATIVE WOMEN

Social, economic, and cultural barriers limit the ability of many American Indians/Alaska Natives (AI/AN) young women to receive accurate and adequate information on preventing HIV and other sexually transmitted infections (STI)s. Young native women need culturally competent, affordable services which build on their assets. Additionally, there is a striking lack of research on cultural issues that influence the reproductive and sexual health of American Indians/Alaska Natives, less on AI/AN adolescents, and even less on young American Indian women.

Young AI/AN Women Suffer High Rates of HIV Infection.

Underreporting is a persistent problem; one study in Los Angeles found that 56 percent of AI/AN patients with HIV were racially misclassified. Nevertheless, the CDC estimates that the rate of AIDS diagnoses for American Indian and Alaska Native adults and adolescents is 9.9 per 100,000 persons. This rate is higher than whites and Asians but lower than blacks and Hispanics. Women accounted for 29 percent of these diagnoses.

## FACTORS CONTRIBUTING TO DISPROPORTIONATE HIV RATES

- The majority of HIV positive AI/AN women (66 percent) contract HIV through heterosexual intercourse, while a significant number (33 percent) are infected through injection drug use.

- A lack of access to health care and/or a lack of trust in health care providers and systems may keep AI/AN young women from receiving adequate medical care, including HIV testing and treatment.
- Intimate partner violence against young AI/AN women is all too common and, since condom negotiation is difficult for women in violent relationships, puts them at risk for HIV. Drugs and alcohol are often factors in cases of sexual violence, thereby increasing risks.
- A lack of education about the disease may lead AI/AN young women to still believe it is a "gay white man's disease," suggesting that they are not at risk.
- Tribal members gather regularly from distant locations for large ceremonies; some young people engage in unprotected sexual contact with acquaintances at these ceremonies, greatly increasing their risk of HIV.

What assets can help protect young AI/AN women from negative sexual outcomes?

- Research shows that parental communication and involvement are very important in empowering young AI/AN women to make healthy decisions about sex (that is, to delay first sex and to use condoms and birth control when having sex).
- Self-efficacy (trust and confidence in one's own decisions) is a powerful protective factor for both condom use, and abstaining from sex.
- Those who do well in school are less likely to be sexually active, while for those who are sexually active, valuing academic achievement is still a protective factor against sexual risk behavior.
- Positive native identity and a sense of belonging to a native community are strongly associated with good sexual health outcomes for AI/AN young women. Research shows that female adolescents from families who lived on a reservation and spoke a tribal language have sex for the first time at an older age and are more likely to use condoms than those from families who do

not; while urban-dwelling youth benefit from programs that emphasize a connection to native culture.

**Young AI/NA Women Need Effective, Culturally Specific Interventions**

- Native youth should be included in creating, designing, and implementing programs and policies around sexuality education.
- Many opportunities exist for involving native youth and empowering them to teach their peers; successful approaches have included:
  - o peer education through traditional and contemporary cultural performance activities;
  - o cultural enrichment and community involvement for young people; programs focused in athletics or the arts;
  - o and programs that emphasized the individual's importance in helping the whole community.
- Young native women need comprehensive sexual education, including information about both contraception and condoms. An important step is integrating condoms into Native cultures. For instance, one researcher suggests packaging the condoms discreetly, so that AI/AN young people feel more comfortable receiving them, and distributing them at powwows and other ceremonies, clinics, and social events.
- Young AI/AN women need access to confidential, culturally competent health care.

**SAVING INDIAN WOMEN FROM HIV/AIDS**

Chatterjee's article provides an overview of the impact of HIV/AIDS in India where the combination of HIV/AIDS and gender bias create a particularly difficult situation for women. The epidemic is occurring where "millions of women remain trapped in a social-cultural context that denies them information, medical treatment, and protection against unsafe sex, which accounts for 85% of HIV infections in the country."

Chatterjee's article seeks to bring attention to World AIDS Day held December 1, 2004. She offers a story of Geeta, a thirty year old woman, who contracts HIV/AIDS from her husband. When it is clear that she's ill, her husband refuses to help her get the medical attention she needs. When he realises she has AIDS, he throws her, and their 8 year daughter out of the house. According to Chatterjee, a newly formed Network of HIV-positive People (Haryana), is accepting members who share the same story. So far there are 80 members, "half of whom are widows and married women who contracted HIV from their husband, and then were blamed, shamed and finally thrown out of their family homes."

Geeta's story helps illustrate Chataterjee's point of just how vulnerable women are. India's Ministry of Health and Family Welfare forecast an increase in the levels of HIV infection "among Indian women, who, largely monogamous themselves, have virtually no control over their husbands' sexual behaviour."

According to the article, brochures providing information about Voluntary Counselling and Testing Centre (VCTCs) and Prevention of Parent to Child Transmission of HIV/AIDS [PPTCTs] are generally found in district hospitals and the offices of non-governmental organisations and international agencies. "They are not reaching village primary health centres." Even if this information were to reach its target market, the messages would need to be "very simple" while avoiding technical terms and meaningless acronyms.

According to Lakshman Singh, President of the Network, if the Network is to be effective in reaching people, it must first reach people with a general health discussion that gradually moves to the subject of sexually transmitted diseases and HIV/AIDS.

## INDIA

India is facing urgent predictions of an HIV explosion, especially among women, for whom currently available prevention strategies (abstinence, mutual monogamy, and male condom use) may not be realistic options. Clearly, woman-controlled barrier methods and microbicides would contribute to Indian women's ability to protect themselves from HIV and other STIs. Because barrier methods also provide dual-protection, preventing both infection and unwanted pregnancy, they are of interest to family planning providers and consumers in India.

India has advanced capabilities in research, manufacture, marketing and distribution of contraceptive and other medical technologies. An Indian company will soon begin distributing a locally manufactured version of the 'Reality' female condom, and other female-initiated barrier methods are likely to be produced and piloted there. Clinical trials of microbicides are also underway in India. In addition, Indian NGOs have a strong history of working in reproductive health and rights, and more and more are looking at issues of HIV and AIDS from a rights-based framework. These combined factors make a compelling case for India to become a leader in advancing the development and introduction of HIV prevention methods for women.

The Global Campaign has worked formally with partners in India since February 2001, the Indian Network of NGOs working on HIV and AIDS (IN-N) invited us to present a technical paper at their 5th National Convention in Ahmedabad. IN-N then incorporated awareness-raising and advocacy for prevention options for women into their agenda. Led by the Gujarat AIDS Awareness Project (GAP), several of the Networks' member organisations have become active partners in the Global Campaign's activities, both in India and internationally

## INDIAN SCENARIO

This feature is the first in a series of articles reviewing the state of HIV around the world. While HIV strikes people and populations all over the world, how it impacts each area, each population, and each culture can be very different. This article takes a look at a part of the world hit very hard by the HIV epidemic. A country of more than a billion people with millions living with HIV. HIV Around the World takes us to India.

### *India-Demographics*

Here are some facts about India:

- located in South Asia

- seventh largest country geographically, and the second most populous country in the world
- approximately 1.1 billion people
- four major religions-Hinduism, Buddhism, Jainism, and Sikhism
- while India has the fourth-largest and the second-fastest growing economy in the world, the country still has very high levels of poverty, environmental pollution, disease, and malnutrition.

In some of the urban and more populous areas, there are some primary health care centers that offer quality health care and research.

However, the population growth of India has outpaced the growth of the health care industry, resulting in shortages of health care facilities and qualified health care professionals, especially in rural areas. India's health care system is overseen by the Ministry of Health and Family Welfare.

## THE STATUS OF HIV AND HIV CARE

Here are some facts about HIV in India:

- HIV emerged as a problem in India almost a decade later than the rest of the world.
- HIV rates skyrocketed in the 1990's and continues today. In fact, India has the highest population of people living with HIV anywhere in the world.
- At first, HIV was isolated to high-risk populations such as sex workers and the country's huge truck driver force. Today, all sectors of India's population is affected.
- It is estimated that in 1990 there were approximately 200,000 people infected with HIV in India. By 2003 that number had climbed to 5.1 million. Currently, it's estimated that between 5.2 and 5.7 million people are living with HIV in the country.
- HIV prevalence estimates vary depending on who you talk to. The World Health Organization (WHO) reports that India's HIV prevalence is on the rise with 5.7 million

people living with HIV, while India's National AIDS Prevention and Control Policy (NACO) says the spread of HIV is 5.2 million and slowing down.

**Who's Infected?:** As was stated earlier, HIV has progressed from a disease found in only the highest-risk population to one found in all segments of the Indian population, be it men, women, rich, poor, urban or rural. Populations thought at one time to be low risk are now being infected, as are high-risk groups. Some groups are being infected at a higher rate than others, however. For instance, women are being infected by way of heterosexual transmission at an alarming rate. Women now make up about 39 percent of those people living with HIV. Most are being infected by husbands or boyfriends who have multiple sexual partners, many of whom are HIV infected and do not know it. Here are some facts about those populations considered to have the highest risk of acquiring HIV.

- *Sex Workers:* Because of widespread poverty throughout India, women often resort to prostitution as a means of making money for their families. Others are forced into sex work due to an underground of violence and disrespect toward women. Finally, women involved in marital break-ups will often begin prostituting themselves as a means of surviving financially after being left with children to feed and a household to support. In some areas of India, it's estimated that one in every two sex workers are HIV infected, many not knowing it.
- *IV Drug Use (IVDU):* The recreational use of drugs often overlaps with the sex trade. While IVDU seems to be worse in the northeastern parts of India, it is common throughout the country. Many attribute the widespread problem of IVDU and HIV to government policies that do not support HIV prevention and risk reduction among IV drug users. Because IVDU is a crime and is consistently enforced and prosecuted, getting prevention messages to users is very difficult. There have been instances of prevention workers themselves being arrested while trying to help and educate IV drug users. Official estimates actually report the HIV prevalence

among IV drug users to have gone down from 13 percent in 2003 to 10 percent in 2005.

- *Truck Drivers:* India's economy depends a great deal on its very large trucking network across the country. While truckers help move goods and services throughout India, they also contribute a great deal to the huge HIV population and the spread of HIV from one area of India to another. Truckers will pick-up sex workers along their route, engage in unprotected sex activity and then drop off the sex worker at the trucker's next stop along the route. This has contributed to the spread of HIV from urban areas into the rural towns and villages. The most damaging fact about truckers and their use of sex workers is that neither party knows they are infected.
- *Men Having Sex with Men:* There is a high degree of stigma associated with homosexuality in India. In fact, homosexuality has been criminalized, making HIV education and surveillance very difficult. Outreach workers are often harassed and even arrested for "promoting homosexuality." It's estimated that 42 percent of all men who have sex with men are also married, fueling the increasing HIV infection rate among women of India.
- *Migrant Workers:* As is the case in the United States, migrant workers in India are very transient and mobile, moving from town to town wherever the work takes them. Unfortunately, they take their risky behavior along with them, fueling the spread of HIV throughout India. While there are attempts at HIV education, the variety of languages, dialects, and cultures makes HIV education very difficult.

## HIV AROUND THE WORLD-INDIA

The national government of India has given the responsibility for HIV prevention and education to the individual states across the country. Each state has its own AIDS Prevention and Control Society that are collectively guided by the National AIDS Prevention and Control Society (NACO). India has devoted US$2.5 billion, however, barriers at the state level such as language and dialect differences make a national prevention and education plan very difficult.

There is a huge push to use condoms. Condom machines are being placed in colleges, roadside rest areas, restaurants, gas stations, and along truck routes in an effort to promote and increase condom use. However, the stigma surrounding condom use remains, impeding the process.

In response, national celebrities are publicly promoting condom use in an effort to remove stigmas surrounding condom use. In an effort to further HIV education, teachers and peer educators are being trained in order to increase the availability and ease of access to HIV education.

## HIV Testing

Currently, India's official stance on HIV testing is that it is voluntary. However, there is a high incidence of "forced testing," especially among patients preparing to have surgery. Unfortunately, those testing positive for HIV most often will have their surgery cancelled by the surgeon. Because of HIV stigmas, many people are afraid to get tested for fear of retribution if they are found to be infected. To make matters worse, a very high percentage of health care workers are not very HIV aware, which only contributes to the stigmas and prejudices.

## HIV Treatment

India is home to some of the largest distributors of HIV medications in the world. Ironically, only about seven percent of those Indian citizens that need HIV medications can access them. The high rate of poverty in the country makes it very difficult if not impossible for most people to get HIV drug regimens.

There are attempts to improve access to HIV drugs. One such initiative involves the use of a single dose of the HIV medication Nevirapine to help decrease the incidence of HIV transmission from a mother to her unborn child. Unfortunately, the prevalent stigmas surrounding HIV cause some pregnant women to avoid any HIV medication for fear of what would happen if her HIV diagnosis was made public.

## SHAII CAMPAIGN FOR ORPHANS AND VULNERABLE CHILDREN

The number of children in India orphaned and left vulnerable by AIDS is approaching two million. The World Bank has dubbed India as being the epicenter of the AIDS orphan crisis because it has the largest number of AIDS orphans in the world. According to the UNAIDS 2006 AIDS epidemic update, of the 5.7 million people estimated to be living with HIV (the highest in the world), at least 250,000 are children. In 2005 alone-60,000 children died of AIDS and 75,000 new pediatric cases were reported. While India has emerged as being the leading producer of generic medicines, less than 10% of children in dire need of treatment are receiving it. Despite this, orphans and vulnerable children (OVC) have remained the forgotten face of the AIDS pandemic in India.

## ACCESS TO TREATMENT AND MEDICINES

Children infected with HIV have very little access to antiretroviral treatment (ART) and essential medicines that can dramatically slow down the spread of the virus in the body. Of the 70,000 children in dire need of treatment, only 1,048 of them are getting it. In cases where children are receiving treatment, they do not have access to pediatric formulations of the drug. Instead, pills that are given to adult AIDS patients are broken into smaller pieces and given to infected children. Many times, receiving the incorrect dosage of medicine, leads to the death of the child. Although the WHO has provided guidelines for the treatment of infants and children infected with HIV, India has yet to develop and implement these guidelines and secure pediatric formulations of ARVs that can increase the life span by 10-15 years for HIV/AIDS children and allow them to live until adolescence or adulthood. Furthermore, as stated by the WHO and other such institutions, the key to stopping pediatric AIDS is to prevent mother-to-child transmission (MTCT). Although there are medicines that can help prevent MTCT, less than 4% of pregnant Indian women receive these medicines or are given consultations to explain the significance of ART. Due to lack of access to essential medicines, over 60,000 HIV positive births occur per year in India.

SHAII has already begun spearheading a campaign to secure pediatric formulations of AIDS drugs. For example, when the combination liquid pediatric formulations were not being distributed through government programs, SHAII worked extensively with the Global AIDS Alliance to bring attention to pediatric guidelines and medicines in India. An action alert was issued to demand formulation of pediatric guidelines and treatment for children living with HIV/AIDS. In addition to the SHAII data base of more than 3000 people, the action alert was circulated on other list-serves, requesting people to send letters to Indian officials to provide pediatric formulation through government supported programs.

As a result of SHAII's advocacy efforts, wide positive response was evoked in India. Many international and Indian organizations commended SHAII on taking the initiative on a much needed advocacy issue. SHAII received positive responses from Indian officials as well. Additionally, in collaboration with GAA, SHAII produced reading materials for public education and communicated with Indian officials to push for the provision of the pediatric drug. SHAII was covered by a wide range of Indian newspapers, such as The Hindu, and The Frontline for its campaign on access to medicines for OVCs.

During the 2001 UN General Assembly Special Session (UNGASS) on HIV/AIDS, world leaders came together to formulate goals and commitments towards the HIV/AIDS pandemic that is sweeping through their countries. The Indian government made major commitments to not only reduce HIV/AIDS prevalence by 25% and increase access to health care for women from 5% to 20%, but also to develop protocols for the care and treatment of the OVC. Unfortunately, the Indian government failed to meet either one of the goals that they themselves had set. When world leaders met again at the 2006 UNGASS on HIV/AIDS to assess their accomplishments, SHAII's public and media advocacy drew widespread attention to the Indian government's inability to fulfill its commitments of 2001 UNGASS goals and the need for pediatric guidelines for orphans and vulnerable children due to HIV/AIDS. SHAII successfully organized a campaign for the rights of the OVC that galvanized India's National AIDS Control Organization (NACO) into announcing provision of pediatric medications through government programs. NACO also conceded to make orphans and vulnerable children a greater priority of the NACP-III, part three of their National AIDS Control Program that will begin this year.

SHAII's campaign for the OVC, specifically in securing pediatric drug formulations and treatment guidelines, is intertwined with its campaign to protect global access to medicines. While India is the leading producer of generic medicines, the government is considering making TRIPS-plus amendments to its Drug and Cosmetics Act that may severely reduce access to affordable generic pediatric formulations of AIDS medicines due to pressure by the U.S. and multinational pharmaceutical companies. Recognizing the adverse affects these amendments may have on increasing access to treatment and medicines for OVCs, SHAII has maintained leadership in advocating against these amendments and bringing international attention to the negative impacts they may have on developing countries that import medicines from Indian generic companies. For more information, click here.

Recently, on World AIDS Day 2006, when India declared a public partnership with the Clinton foundation to provide 62 countries with low cost pediatric formulations of AIDS drugs and to expand its own treatment outreach for children living with HIV, SHAII immediately responded to the consequences of implementing the program without policies in tact for the treatment, care and protection of OVCs. "Although a great initiative", as stated by Dr. Gupta, director and founder of The Stop HIV/AIDS in India Initiative (SHAII), "with less than 100 physicians trained to treat India's more than 250,000 children living with HIV/AIDS, adopting a narrow and target-based approach to increase treatment access from 1,048 to 10,000 children in four months without a strong policy framework and guidelines may prove to be counterproductive." Click here for SHAII press release.

## Care and Protection of OVC Rights

India's HIV/AIDS pandemic is particular due to the intensity of wide-spread stigma that is embedded within Indian society that have resulted in human rights violations against innocent children. The stigma, ignorance and apprehension surrounding HIV/AIDS has led to discriminatory actions taken against children, such as being kicked out of educational institutions, rejected from orphanages, denied treatment from doctors and hospitals, and alienated from both the family and community. These children have no choice but to become "street children"- being left completely exposed to criminal activities, drug trafficking, sex trade, and child labor.

A major challenge to stopping pediatric AIDS is the low status given to women in Indian society, specifically the girl-child. Girls are less likely to receive aid, and are more vulnerable to sexual exploitation due to their disadvantaged socio-cultural status. They are the first to be taken out of schools and must take up the role of care-giver to their siblings if a parent dies. In order to care for their families, the girl-child (ranging from age 7-15) becomes exposed to prostitution and the sex trade, making her more likely to contract HIV.

A critical aspect of SHAII's OVC campaign is its promotion of the status and rights of the girl-child through our project addressing female feticide. Female feticide is when a mother decides to get an abortion upon determination of the female sex status of her fetus. Thus, female feticide is an indicator of the low status associated with the girl child. In India, there are very few organizations working on female feticide and very little information is available on the issue. Due to social pressures and norms, the mother is indirectly forced to make the decision to abort her female fetus. Additionally, the laws that address the issue of female feticide are not strong and do not prosecute those involved. Essentially, the sex determination law in India is non-functional and of the cases involving female feticide, none have been prosecuted. The number of cases reported to the human rights commission and the Indian census are also not the same (735 and ~874 respectively).

This project will address female feticide by increasing social awareness through public education; creating social support systems for women and the girl child; promoting the adoption and education of the girl child through E-advocacy and scholarship programs; engaging women leadership and forming self-help groups; and analyzing, developing and implementing policies at the grassroots community and state levels. By tackling female feticide, this project simultaneously increases access to treatment and medicines for gild children and women affected by HIV/AIDS via the promotion of the girl child and empowering women.

SHAII's OVC campaign is a holistic model designed to fight HIV/AIDS in India at various levels and focuses on increasing visibility to bring about policy changes for the treatment, care and protection of the OVC. Specifically, SHAII's objective is:

To increase attention, commitment and funding to OVC issues.

To stimulate India to develop policies to protect and promote OVC rights, including those of the girl child.

To increase access to care, treatment and medicines for OVC affected by HIV/AIDS.

Our strength lies within our strategy. Through public education, grassroots and coalition building, and public advocacy, we want to activate the NRI community simultaneously with the international health and human rights sector in and outside of India, in order to provide continuous scrutiny and pressure over pediatric healthcare policy development and implementation in India.

India is a vast, diverse and populous country with significant social, economic and cultural disparities within-and between-the country's different regions.

In 2001, India was home to one-sixth of the world's population: some 1,032 million people. Of these, over 35% live on less than US$1 a day. While poverty affects both men and women, it is India's women-particularly dalits, those from the lowest caste, and women from tribal communities-who suffer most.

India's progressive Constitution attempts to address this marginalisation through policies of positive discrimination, often 'reserving' public sector and government jobs for those from scheduled castes and tribes. However, such policies are neither well received by some sections of India's wider population, nor have they yet impacted significantly on the health, education and income of marginalised communities.

Strong social, cultural and religious traditions continue to hinder women's progress towards full and active participation in their own lives, within their families, their communities and their country. For many of India's women, there is a wide disparity between their country's progressive reforms and their daily experience.

Fact File:

- Population: 1,032 million (at 2001)
- Of these, 531 million are women
- 62% of women are illiterate
- India has the 2nd highest rate of HIV/AIDS in the world
- 5.1 million Indians are infected
- 38% of those living with HIV are women
- For every 1000 boy babies born in the country there were only 933 female infants
- Neglect of girl babies and female foeticide exists in 27 of India's 32 states
- One woman dies every 5 minutes in childbirth
- Over 100,000 woman die each year from pregnancy-related causes
- More than 15,000 women every year are victims of dowry-related violence

## EXPLORATIONS IN THE CULTURAL HISTORY OF AIDS

### HIV/AIDS: A Threat to Indian Feminism

In this global world HIV/AIDS is not just merely a health issue. It is a multifaceted issue which cannot be reduced to medical terminology only. HIV/AIDS is very much a social/ human problem in Developing Countries like India.

The research shows that 90% of the women who are living with HIV/AIDS are married women and are in monogamous relationships. There are estimated 2 million women infected by

HIV in India that is why the research groups in India are now calling AIDS as 'women disease'. In the majority of cases, the woman would not have even known about the possibility of contracting the disease through sexual relations with her husband/partner. Even if she knew and was aware of the precautions that ought to be taken, she would not have been in a position to insist.

In India the major cause of turning of HIV/AIDS into an epidemic is due to gender inequality. Secondly, the Indian social structure is masculine dominated and the patriarch of the family whether nuclear or joint family are males and women are just their subservient which makes them more vulnerable to this disease. The major transmitter of HIV are their male partners.

The dearth of empirically derived knowledge about sexual behaviour has unfortunately given rise to host of myths and unfounded stereotypes about sex which resulted in rapid increase of HIV cases. Besides sex, the practice of tattooing is common in rural and tribal areas to both men and women. They use same needle for pricking. This very practice is becoming a means of transmission of HIV now a days as tattooing is must for rural and tribal women. However, the research shows that women are least affected by HIV in the cases of blood transfusion as in most hospitals blood test is mandatory.

Women infected with these disease are either blamed or not recognised as potential patients.The consequence can be delayed diagnosis and treatment, stigmatization, loss of income and violation and human rights. Social and psychological burdens on women are more than men. These include problems related to pregnancy and motherhood, rejection of marital partner, loss of security etc. In many cases women have increased risk to HIV because they are from lower strata of society and are totally economically depended on their male partners. Preventive strategies are taken by policy-makers.

In the state of Andhra Pradesh, the government has made a law that before marriage both male and female have to take HIV tests. Besides government, non-governmental organizations and other agencies have designed innovative schemes to educate women so that the transmission of this deadly disease can be avoided within the parameters of Indian social structure. My paper will explain how political, social and economic impact on Indian women by HIV/AIDS epidemic and the crusade taken by government, various agencies and organizations against this dreaded virus.

## HIV/AIDS MOTHER-TO-CHILD TRANSMISSION IN INDIA: SOCIAL AND CULTURAL FACTORS

**Purpose:** To bring preliminary understanding of the cultural and social factors of the HIV/AIDS mother to child transmission in India Experimental method: Multidisciplinary and multicentric field researches in social anthropology and in psycho-sociology in Tamil Nadu (South India) developed in French Institute of Pondicherry (2002-2004), and Indo-French round-table on the subject with Indian and French medical specialists social scientists (2002).

**Results and Conclusions:** Cultural and social factors acting in MTCT appear as a multifactorial issue, not reduced to the behavioural aspects. A number of factors can be identified in the Indian health system. The public governmental health policy has included prevention of HIV/AIDS epidemic as a priority. But in fact, identification and testing of HIV of Indian women are not always followed by further proper information and counselling. Preventing or curing treatment and proper medical monitoring are lacking in the public sector. Medical professionals are meeting a number of difficulties to face HIV-positive people: reaction of stigmatization, fear of transmission, lack of skills. In private medical system, the financial aspects bring inequalities to the accessibility of treatment and care. NGOs are also acting but they are not always involved in the proper networking to get information and training. The local applications of international recommendations raise a number of difficulties: international epidemiology results/local realities towards habits of breast-feeding, changes of recommendations for breast-feeding/difficulties of medical professional to deal with, international standardised concept of 'counselling'/'popular' concept of 'counselling' even among medical professionals, accessibility of proper training for medical professionals and for those acting in prevention, etc. The behavioural aspects of prevention (specially style of breast-feeding or alternative feeding) need to be enlarged to the social and cultural dynamics of the Indian society: social valorization of breast-feeding, social, sexual and biological vulnerable status of women and girls, stigmatization and exclusion of HIV-positive people, of divorcee, of widows, couple, family and community dimensions of women behaviours and decisions, medical pluralism and diversity of health seeking behaviours, of representations of HIV/AIDS and of its transmission and of its way of prevention, etc.

## NOTHING POSITIVE-AIDS AND THE INDIAN WOMAN

The fact that over 19 lakh women in India are living with HIV AIDS is setting off alarm bells in the Indian medical fraternity-especially since more than 90 percent of these are married women in monogamous relationships...

- More married women in India are at risk of getting AIDS than sex workers
- India is about to be hit by the worst AIDS epidemic in the world
- Research groups are now calling AIDS in India 'a woman's disease'

It is easy to misjudge the challenge of HIV/AIDS. Rarely perceived as a major public health issue in India, AIDS has taken on nightmarish proportions in recent years. The large population, low literacy and even lower levels of awareness has made AIDS one of the most challenging public health problems ever faced by the country.

The rising number of women (over 1.9 million at the last count) afflicted with AIDS is setting off alarm bells in the Indian medical fraternity-especially since more than 90 percent of these are married women and are in a monogamous relationship.

In the light of these statistics, Breakthrough, a human rights organisation has launched a media campaign titled What Kind Of Man Are You? The campaign highlights the rising incidence of married women infected by the AIDS virus by their husbands.

## Crusade Against AIDS

As part of the crusade against AIDS, popular television stars Mandira Bedi and Samir Soni have joined hands with Breakthrough and both feature in a music video, Maati sung by Shubha Mudgal, Maati talks about a pregnant woman who discovers she is HIV positive because of her husband's promiscuity.

Apart from this, Breakthrough has been organizing various workshops to provide sex education to the general public. It also has an SMS facility through which people's queries are answered, informing them about the treatment and care for the infected.

The organisation has also launched an intensive multimedia campaign to focus public attention on the growing problem of HIV AIDS. The message is being conveyed through music videos, eye catching advertisements in newspapers, radio and television that are being directed by renowned adman Prasun Joshi. The different visuals have the same theme-a woman asking her husband to protect her by using a condom.

The campaign aims to empower women in an exceedingly patriarchal society, enabling them to discuss sexuality freely with their husbands and encouraging the use of condoms among men.

## Negotiating Safe Sex

According to Mallika Dutt, founder and executive director Breakthrough, "It's a challenge for any woman to negotiate safe sex with her husband. Many times the request for a condom may be interpreted as an accusation of promiscuity against the husband. Our campaign helps married women to understand the need for safe sex and how to voice their opinion."

Both Sameer Soni and Mandira Bedi feel that the responsibility and the guilt that a man feels on infecting his innocent wife, is brought out beautifully in the video, directed by Arjun Bali.. "The fact that television and music are so popular with the masses will help spread the message much faster in a populated country like India, than workshops and prevention measures targeting small groups of people," says

Soni. Until recently HIV education programmes targeted only the high-risk population such as truck drivers, drug users and sex workers but the reality is that an increasing number of married women are at risk. They are ignorant about the dangers they face and hence are easy targets of infection.

Most Indian women are completely uninformed about sex and sexual health practices at the time of marriage. Under great pressure to produce children (particularly sons), the use of condoms and other contraceptives does not arise. The low economic and social status of women renders them unable to have much of a say in sex and thus, they cannot suggest the use of a condom which in turn can lead to their becoming infected with the HIV virus.

Cultural practices and outdated beliefs still plague the Indian society and there is rampant discrimination against women. A woman is labelled "immoral and loose" if detected with the deadly virus. Subjected to ill treatment and isolation of the worst kind, these women are faced with no family support, loss of job opportunities and an extremely low economic status.

Worse, there is lack of access to treatment and medical facilities for these women.

Besides they can also be subject to increased violence. Voiceless, disgraced and ostracized, these women sometimes end up being branded as untouchables or worse being killed by their own family members

## Preventive Measures

In India sex is rarely discussed openly. However it is important to educate and inform the people. According to many health experts, the future course of AIDS in Asia will be set by India's example. Sex education in schools to promote the magnitude of safe sex is essential. Yet over 42 percent of boys and 69 percent of girls of 15 years and older do not go to school. To educate them mass media drives and sex education workshops for the general public are essential.

Allopathic medicines like AZT used in combination with other drugs form the main treatment for AIDS related diseases. Also early diagnosis and effective treatment can help in prolonging life expectancy. Research is currently underway for a cure and to develop effective and cheaper female condoms that will put the power of protection against HIV in the woman's hands. But until then the only way to contain the spread of the disease is cooperation by the male partner.

Says Mallika Dutt, "India needs to follow the example of Brazil in aggressively pursuing AIDS prevention and treatment as the country is on the edge of a pandemic that might make India resemble one of those African nations where one in three people is afflicted with the deadly HIV AIDS virus.

Between 5.5 and 6 million people in South Asia are living with HIV and AIDS.

Large concentrated epidemics among high risk groups, including injecting drug users, men who have sex with men, and sex workers and their clients, are driving the HIV epidemic in South Asia.

HIV prevalence among these often vulnerable and marginalized groups is high throughout the region and rapidly increasing in some places.

In India alone more than 5 million people are estimated to be living with HIV and AIDS. India's HIV epidemic is highly heterogeneous and appears to be stable or diminishing in some parts of the country while growing in others. The majority of reported HIV infections are concentrated in six states where HIV prevalence is, on average, 4-5 times higher than in other states.

These include the Mumbai-Karnataka corridor, the Nagpur area of Maharashtra, the Nammakkal district of Tamil Nadu, coastal Andhra Pradesh, and parts of Manipur and Nagaland. Recent data suggest that high levels of condom use in the context of sex work may have played a role in reducing HIV prevalence among young women in some southern Indian states, but not in north India. Still, enhanced efforts are needed to sustain and effectively reach high-risk groups.

Women account for a growing proportion of people living with HIV in India-particularly in rural areas. A large proportion of women with HIV appear to have acquired the virus from regular partners who were infected during paid sex. Although HIV prevention efforts targeting sex workers and their partners are being implemented, the law enforcement context of sex work often acts as a barrier.

In other countries in the region, such as Bangladesh, Nepal, Pakistan and Sri Lanka HIV prevalence is low among the general population but significantly higher among those who engage in high-risk behaviors, such as injecting drugs with contaminated needles and engaging in the selling and buying of sex. These concentrated epidemics are extensive and affect a large proportion of vulnerable populations at high risk. As a result, HIV is spreading rapidly in some parts of the region.

Significant structural and socioeconomic factors across the region put many people at risk of HIV infection:

- More than 35% of the population lives below the poverty line
- Low levels of literacy
- Porous borders
- Rural to urban and intrastate migration of male populations
- Trafficking of women and girls into prostitution
- Stigma related to sex, sexuality and HIV
- Structured commercial sex and casual sex with non-regular partners
- Male resistance to condom use
- High prevalence of sexually transmitted infections (STIs)
- Low status of women, leading to an inability to negotiate safe sex.

## The World Bank Response

In response to these risk factors, the World Bank in South Asia has focused on mobilizing countries to improve and accelerate their response to HIV and AIDS.

The World Bank has supported national efforts to slow the spread of HIV since the first India project in 1992, and has committed US$380 million to support national programs to date.

The main components of these projects are surveillance, monitoring and evaluation, targeted interventions for vulnerable populations, blood safety, efforts aimed at reducing stigma among the general population, and strengthening public and private institutions for a multi-sector response.

In addition, the Bank has undertaken analytical work, including AIDS in South Asia: Understanding and Responding to a Heterogeneous Epidemic (a synthesis of the epidemiology of HIV in the region) and a study on costing of antiretrovirals in India. This work will help to inform policy and evidence-based decision making.

# 9

# Time Line of AIDS

**1958**

- A 25-year-old printer from England named David Carr, who had served in the Royal Navy between 1955 and 1957, contracts a series of mysterious ailments including Pneumocystis carinii. He dies early the next year (1959). In 1990, tests by a hospital in Manchester reveal HIV in Carr's tissue samples, and he is briefly recognized as the first known AIDS death. Subsequent, more sophisticated testing at the Aaron Diamond AIDS Research Center at New York University Medical School reveals the HIV to have been a laboratory contaminant.

**1959**

- The first known case of HIV in a human occurs in a person who died in the Congo, seemingly later confirmed as having HIV infection from his preserved blood samples (Zhu et al., 1998). However, according to the authors of the 1959 discovery, they never found, nor alleged to have found, HIV, or anything like a full virus. According to these authors, even "attempts to amplify HIV-1 fragments of >300 base pairs (bp) were unsuccessful,... However, after numerous attempts, four shorter sequences were obtained" that only represented small portions of two of the six genes of the complete AIDS virus. Citation: Zhu T, Korber BT, Nahmias AJ, Hooper E, Sharp PM and Ho DD. An African HIV-1 sequence from 1959 and implications for the origin of the epidemic.

- In New York City, a 49-year-old Haitian-born shipping clerk dies of Pneumocystis carinii pneumonia, a disease closely associated with AIDS victims. Dr. Gordon Hennigar, who performed the postmortem examination of the man's body, has been quoted in numerous publications saying that he believes the man probably had AIDS.

**1969**

- A St. Louis teenager, identified only as Robert R., dies of an illness that baffles his doctors. Eighteen years later, molecular biologists at Tulane University in New Orleans test samples of his remains and find the virus that causes AIDS. source New York Times.

**1975**

- The first reports of wasting and other symptoms, later determined to be AIDS, are reported in residents of Africa.

**1976**

- Norwegian sailor Arvid Noe dies; it is later determined that he contracted HIV/AIDS in Africa during the early 1960s.

**1977**

- Danish physician Grethe Rask dies of AIDS contracted in Africa.
- A San Francisco prostitute gives birth to the first of three children who would later be diagnosed with AIDS, and whose blood, when tested after their deaths, would reveal HIV infection. The mother would herself die of AIDS in May 1987. She was clearly infected as early as 1977 and perhaps as early as 1976, when the current epidemic is believed to have reached the United States.

**1978**

- A Portuguese man known as Senhor Jose dies; he will later be confirmed as the first known infection of

HIV-2. He was believed to have been exposed to the disease in Guinea-Bissau in 1966.

**1980**

- April 24, San Francisco resident Ken Horne, the first AIDS case in the United States to be recognized at the time, is reported to Center for Disease Control with Kaposi's sarcoma. He was also suffering from Cryptococcus at the time.
- On October 31, French-Canadian flight attendant Gaetan Dugas pays his first known visit to New York City bathhouses. He would later be deemed "Patient Zero" for his apparent connection to many early cases of AIDS in the United States.

**1981**

- January 15, Nick Rock becomes the first known AIDS death in New York City.
- May 18, Dr. Lawrence Mass becomes the first journalist in the world to write about the epidemic, in the "New York Native," a gay newspaper. A gay tipster overheard his physician mention that some gay men were being treated in intensive-care units in New York City for a strange pneumonia. "Disease Rumors Largely Unfounded" was the headline on Mass's article. Mass repeated a New York City public-health official's claims that there was no wave of disease sweeping through the gay community. At this point, however, the CDC had been gathering information for about a month on the outbreak that Mass's source was dismissing.
- June 5, CDC reports a cluster of Pneumocystis pneumonia in five gay male drug users in Los Angeles.
- July 4, CDC reports clusters of Kaposi's sarcoma and Pneumocystis pneumonia among gay men in California and New York City.

**1982**

- June 18, CDC MMWR 1982 31(23);305-7

"Exposure to some substance (rather than an infectious agent) may eventually lead to immunodeficiency among a subset of the homosexual male population that shares a particular style of life. For example, Marmor et al. recently reported that exposure to amyl nitrite was associated with an increased risk of KS in New York City. Exposure to inhalant sexual stimulants, central-nervous-system stimulants, and a variety of other "street" drugs was common among males belonging to the cluster of cases of KS and PCP in Los Angeles and Orange counties."

- July 9, CDC reports a cluster of opportunistic infections and Kaposi's sarcoma among Haitians recently entering the United States.
- July 27, The term AIDS (for acquired immune deficiency syndrome) is proposed at a meeting in Washington of gay-community leaders, federal bureaucrats and the Centers for Disease Control and Prevention (CDC)
- September 24, Current Trends Update on Acquired Immune Deficiency Syndrome (AIDS)-United States

  CDC defines a case of AIDS as a disease, at least moderately predictive of a defect in cell-mediated immunity, occurring in a person with no known cause for diminished resistance to that disease. Such diseases include KS, PCP, and serious OOI. [...] Diagnoses are considered to fit the case definition only if based on sufficiently reliable methods (generally histology or culture). Some patients who are considered AIDS cases on the basis of diseases only moderately predictive of cellular immunodeficiency may not actually be immunodeficient and may not be part of the current epidemic.
- December 10, a baby in California becomes ill in the first known case of AIDS from a blood transfusion.

**1983**

- In January, Dr. Francoise Barre, at the Pasteur Institute in Paris, isolates a retrovirus that kills T-cells from the lymph system of a gay AIDS patient. In the following months, she would find it in additional gay and hemophiliac sufferers. This retrovirus would be called by several names, including LAV and HTLV-III before being named HIV in 1986.

- CDC National AIDS Hotline established.
- March, Food and Drug Administration (FDA) issues donor screening guidelines. AIDS high-risk groups should not donate blood/plasma products.
- Australia has first death from AIDS in Melbourne, the Hawke Labor government invests a significant campaign that gave Australia one of the lowest infection rates in the World.

**1984**

- April 23, U.S. Health and Human Services Secretary Margaret Heckler announces at a press conference that an American scientist, Dr. Robert Gallo, has discovered the probable cause of AIDS: the retrovirus subsequently named human immunodeficiency virus or HIV in 1986. She also declares that a vaccine will be available within two years.
- September 6, first performance at Theatre Rhinoceros in San Francisco of The AIDS Show which runs for two years and is the subject of a 1986 documentary film of the same name.

**1985**

- March 2, FDA approves first AIDS antibody screening tests for use on all donated blood and plasma intended for transfusion.
- October 2, Rock Hudson, the first American celebrity to publicly admit having AIDS, dies of the disease.
- October, a conference of public health officials including representatives of the Centers for Disease Control and World Health Organisation meet in Bangui and define AIDS in Africa as "prolonged fevers for a month or more, weight loss of over 10% and prolonged diarrhoea".

**1986**

- HIV (human immunodeficiency virus) is adopted as name of the retrovirus that was first proposed as the cause of AIDS by Luc Montagnier of France, who named it LAV (lymphadenopathy associated virus) and Robert Gallo of the United States, who named it HTLV-III (human T-lymphotropic virus type III)
- January 14, "By 1996, three to five million Americans will be HIV positive and one million will be dead of AIDS"-NIAID Director Anthony Fauci, New York Times

**1987**

- "By 1990 one in five heterosexuals will be dead of AIDS"-Oprah Winfrey.

**1993**

- CDC expands definition of AIDS to include a person with HIV infection and a CD4 cell count below 200. CDC estimates that the expanded definition could increase cases reported in 1993 by approximately 75%.

**1996**

- Robert Gallo's discovery that a natural compound known as chemokines can block HIV and halt the progression of AIDS is hailed by Science magazine as one of that year's most important scientific breakthroughs.

**1997**

- September 2, "The most recent estimate of the number of Americans infected (with HIV), 750,000, is only half the total that government officials used to cite over a decade ago, at a time when experts believed that as many as 1.5 million people carried the virus." article in the Washington Post
- Based on the Bangui definition the WHO's cumulative number of reported AIDS cases from 1980 through 1997 for all of Africa is 620,000. For comparison, the cumulative total of AIDS cases in the USA through 1997 is 641,087.

**1998**

- December 10, International Human Rights Day, Treatment Action Campaign (TAC) is launched to campaign for greater access to HIV treatment for all South Africans, by raising public awareness and understanding about issues surrounding the availability, affordability and use of HIV treatments. TAC campaigns against the view that AIDS is a death sentence.

**1999**

- January 31, studies suggest that a retrovirus, SIVcpz (simian immunodeficiency virus) from the common chimpanzee Pan troglodytes, may have passed to human populations in west equatorial Africa during the twentieth century and developed into various types of HIV.

  F Gao, E Bailes, DL Robertson, Y Chen, CM Rodenburg, SF Michael, LB Cummins, LO Arthur, M Peeters, GM Shaw, PM Sharp and BH Hahn. Origin of HIV-1 in the chimpanzee Pan troglodytes troglodytes. Nature 397, 436-41 (1999).

  RA Weis and RW Wrangham. From Pan to pandemic. Nature 397, 385-6 (1999).

- The role of chemokines in protection from progression of HIV infection to AIDS is changing the medical understanding of AIDS.

**2000**

- WHO estimates between 15% and 20% of new HIV infections worldwide are the result of blood transfusions, where the donors were not screened or inadequately screened for HIV.

**2001**

- September 21, FDA licenses the first nucleic acid test (NAT) systems intended for screening of blood and plasma donors.

**2004**

- January 5, "Individual risk of acquiring HIV and experiencing rapid disease progression is not uniform within populations", says Anthony S. Fauci, M.D., director of NIAID.

**2005**

- January 21, CDC recommends anti-retroviral post-exposure prophylaxis for people exposed to HIV from rapes, accidents or occasional unsafe sex or drug use. This treatment should start no more than 72 hours after a person has been exposed to the virus, and the drugs should be used by patients for 28 days. This emergency drug treatment has been recommended since 1996 for health-care workers accidentally stuck with a needle, splashed in the eye with blood, or exposed in some other way on the job.

**2006**

- June 5th is the 25th anniversary of the first reported AIDS cases.
- November 9th 2006, HIV found in Gorillas, HIV-1 and HIV-2.

# Bibliography


Adrian Burgess: *Psychological Medicine of HIV Infection,* Oxford, New York, Oxford University Press, 1995.

Altman, D.: *AIDS and Security. Health Impacts of Globalization*, Palgrave, MacMillan, 2003.

Ankrah, E.M.: *Knowledge, Attitudes and Practices (KAP) Study for School Health Education: Implications for AIDS Control*, Kampala, Uganda: UNICEF, 1987.

Barbara, Hermie: *Working together against AIDS,* New York, Rosen Pub. Group, 1995.

Bartlett, John G.: *The Guide to Living with HIV Infection, Developed at the Johns Hopkins AIDS Clinic*, Baltimore, Johns Hopkins University Press, 1998.

Bundy D.A.P.: *Helminth Infection. in Disease Control Priorities in Developing Countries*, Oxford University Press, Oxford, 1993.

Catalan, Jose: *Psychological Medicine of HIV Infection,* Oxford, New York, Oxford University Press, 1995.

Crompton, D.W.T., : *Ascariasis and its Prevention and Control*, Taylor & Francis, London, 1989.

Eileen, D.: *Toolkit for HIV Prevention among Mobile Populations in the Greater Mekong Subregion Part two Country Resources*, Melbourne, The Macfarlane Burnet Institute for Medical Reseach, 2002.

Forbes, Anna: *Kids with AIDS,* New York, Rosen Pub. Group's Powerkids Press, 1996.

Fuller, B.: *The Risk of HIV Transmission amongst Youth in Pohnpei*, Melbourne, Monash University, 2001.

Ivana Klines: *Psychological Medicine of HIV Infection,* Oxford, New York, Oxford University Press, 1995.

Joseph, R.: *Outpatient Management of HIV Infection,* St. Louis, Mosby, 1996.

Jussim, Daniel. *AIDS & HIV: Risky Business,* Springfield, N.J., Enslow Publishers, 1997.

Kenneth J.: *AIDS, Fear, and Society: Challenging the Dreaded Disease,* Washington, Taylor & Francis, 1997.

Laura Pinsky: *The Essential AIDS Fact Book,* New York, Pocket Books, 1996.

Nesheim, M.C. : *Ascariasis and its Prevention and Control,* Taylor & Francis, London, 1989.

Paul, Hampton: *HIV Law: a Survival Guide to the Legal System for People living with HIV,* New York, Three Rivers Press, 1997.

Pawlowski, Z.S.: *Ascariasis and its Prevention and Control,* Taylor & Francis, London, 1989.

Powell, Josh: *AIDS and HIV-related Diseases: an Educational Guide for Professionals and the Public,* New York, Insight Books, 1996.

Robert, M.: *AIDS Law in a Nutshell,* St. Paul, West Pub. Co., 1996.

Romeyn, Mary: *Nutrition and HIV: a New Model for Treatment,* San Francisco, Jossey-Bass Publishers, 1998.

Rwabukwali, C.B.: *Knowledge, Attitudes and Practices (KAP) Study for School Health Education: Implications for AIDS Control,* Kampala, Uganda: UNICEF, 1987.

Seth, C.: *Answering your questions about AIDS,* Washington, American Psychological Association, 1996.

Stephenson, L.S.: *The Impact of Helminth Infections on Human Nutrition: Schistosomes and Soil-transmitted Helminths,* Taylor & Francis, London, 1987.

Tonks, Douglas: *Teaching AIDS.* New York, Routledge, 1996.

Virginia, A., and Melissa Gross: *HIV/AIDS Information for Children: a guide to Issues and Resources,* New York, H. W. Wilson Co., 1996.

Warren, K.S.: *Helminth Infection. in Disease Control Priorities in Developing Countries,* Oxford University Press, Oxford, 1993.

# Index

## I



## J



## L



## M



## N



## O

□□□